Letters to My Sisters

An Alzheimer's Journal

Letters

to

My Sisters

An Alzheimer's Journal

Patricia M. Thompson

St. Colman Press

P.O. Box 17634

Rochester, New York 14617

ISBN: 1-4116-5214-2

Library of Congress Control Number: 2005907185

Published by
St. Colman Press
P.O. Box 17634
Rochester, NY 14617

In conjunction with
Lulu Enterprises
3131 RDU Center, Suite 210
Morrisville, NC 27560
Lulu ID#: 166106

Cover photo: Carole, Susan, Virginia and Bea; Lake Tahoe, August 1987

This book is dedicated to my son, David, who had a natural instinct for communicating with his grandmother long before I learned those skills.

And to my husband, Gary, without whose help and approval, I never could have brought my Mother to live with us.

TABLE OF CONTENTS

PREFACE

In August 1989, my Mother came from New Mexico to live with us. We knew she was in the early stages of Alzheimer's Disease and could no longer live alone. In January 1990, I began a letter to my sisters to fill them in on how things were going. As it turned out, this letter was to be the first of a series of letters describing to my sisters, who couldn't be here, the day to day experience of living with Alzheimer's. Although these letters were meant to keep the others up to date on Mom's progress, they also served, over the long term, as journal for me, charting the course of our adventure together.

If you have read my former book, *Alzheimer's and the Workplace*, you'll see there all I have learned over the years about Alzheimer's communication skills. How I wish I had known back in 1989 what I know today. I could have made Mom's life (and mine) so much easier. But you can't go back, nor can you know everything you need to know when you need to know it. Reading back over the time covered in these letters, I'm rather amazed that I handled some situations so badly, some pretty well, and yet we seemed to survive in spite of it.

I have never been well known for my patience – definitely not one of my strong suits. However, Alzheimer's was the ultimate trial of what little patience I have. Alzheimer's is a frightening and overwhelming disease for everyone concerned. Perhaps the most distressing part is knowing the victims are aware of what is happening in the early stages. They may deny, make excuses, look for answers, become depressed, try to hide it, but they KNOW. I often thought it would be easier if these folks could just step into this 'other world' all at once without knowing what they were leaving behind.

My first experience with Alzheimer's occurred in 1977. At that time, we were caring for a foster baby, Matthew, and frequently had my Aunt Therese baby-sit. She was a single lady, my father's sister, and lived with two other maiden aunts, Mary and Anne. All three, but particularly Aunt Therese, had cared for my sisters and myself, our cousins, and subsequently, our children as well.

I mention Matthew in the way of introduction because it was an incident with him that initiated my awareness of Alzheimer's in our family. He was about six months old and Aunt Therese had come to baby-sit one morning. I told her to put him down for a nap around 10:00 a.m. and if he wasn't awake by noon, to wake him and give him lunch. When we returned home mid-afternoon, he was sleeping and she told us she had fed him at 10:00 but had a really hard time keeping him awake till noon.

I didn't think too much about it then, but it was odd for her to get directions confused. A few days later, Aunt Mary invited me out to lunch and advised me not to have Aunt Therese baby-sit any more. She was becoming forgetful and Aunt Mary was concerned about the baby's safety. The baby-sitting ended, but we took the children to visit the Aunts more frequently after that.

Over the following months, random occurrences cropped up which initially we wondered at and commented on, but disregarded since they were isolated and infrequent. For instance, during a shopping trip with my sister, Carole, Aunt Therese bought a scarf for Aunt Mary. About ten minutes after leaving the store, she said she had to get a Christmas gift for Aunt Mary. Carole reminded her that she already had the scarf, but she insisted that no, she had not and became very agitated. Carole finally showed her the scarf and after a while Aunt Therese pretended that she did, indeed, remember. She calmed down then and tried to make a joke of it.

It was perhaps in 1980 or 81, when the incidents were too frequent to be dismissed, that Aunt Mary finally got her to a doctor and was given the diagnosis of 'probable' Alzheimer's Disease ('probable' because there was no definitive test; only the process of elimination, ruling out other causes of dementia).

Aunt Therese had taken an early retirement from her job because she sensed a problem building. After getting lost one day on her way home from church – one block away – she gave up going out by herself. In fact, she wouldn't even get up in the morning unless she heard Aunt Mary already up. In the long term, this was a real blessing, because she maintained a sense of needing help and, therefore, didn't wander as many Alzheimer's victims do. In the last few months she was home, I would take care of her two days a week to give the other Aunts a break. During this time period (fall of 1984), she could tell me stories in detail of her childhood, but yesterday and last week were gone. As she lost the ability to speak properly, she almost gave up speaking altogether as it was frustrating not to be able to find the right words.

In January 1985, Aunt Mary placed her in St. Ann's Nursing Home. It was extremely difficult for everyone, but inevitable. Over the next two years, Aunt Anne never went to visit. One day she said to me, "Some day, I'm going to be just like that." She couldn't bear to face what she believed would be her own future. Aunt Therese died in January 1987. Aunt Anne was admitted to St. Ann's in August of that same year with Alzheimer's.

Of course, one of the side effects of all this was the wonder (fear) for my sisters and cousins and me as to whether we would eventually get Alzheimer's as well. In the course of the previous few years, I had learned a great deal about the disease and particularly looked for any evidence that it is genetic. It had been theorized that in some cases, it is genetic and in others, it appears to be totally random. I remember reading in one article that in those cases where it is believed to be genetic, it is a dominant trait. In other words, one of your parents has to have had it. I was relieved to read this since my father, who died at age 79, had shown no signs of dementia. Little did we know what was around the corner.

CHAPTER 1

An Introduction

Beatrice Evelyn Farnan was born March 6, 1912. (In the early stages of Alzheimer's she would proudly announce, "I can always remember my birthday; it's 3-6-12 – see?") In 1933, she became a wife: Beatrice Farnan Manion. In 1934, she became a mother. In 1947 she became my mother. In 1955, she became a grandmother. In 1982, she became a great-grandmother. In 1989, I became her mother.

My Mother was born in Batavia, New York, the fourth of seven children. She grew up on Pembroke St. in Rochester. I know only a few vignettes about her growing up years. She nearly died during a flu epidemic when she was only 6 or 7 years old. She flunked Ancient History in high school and had to repeat it in summer school. She was in a high school sorority and worked at a country club with her friend (eventually her sister-in-law), Nancy Harris. During the time they worked at the country club, they made a pact to get their hair cut. They both wore it quite long at that time. They nervously waited for the hair stylist, and when she called them in, Mom insisted Nan go first. After she came back with dramatically shorter hair, Mom backed out and fled the salon with her long hair intact. Aunt Nan tells that story to this very day. She was engaged to Mom's brother, Kernan, at the time and he was horrified to see her short hair. I don't think she ever got a short haircut again. At 18, Mom took off on a joy ride with a couple of fellows to St. Bonaventure in Olean, NY. They got stopped for speeding, brought before a judge and nearly thrown in jail. The fine was $55; among the three of them, they only had $8. As it happened, one of the two boys was the son of the Chief of Police in Rochester. They called him to rescue them and, luckily, Chief Doyle never reported the incident to Mom's parents.

In September of 1932, Mom was the maid-of-honor at her sister's wedding. It was there she met George Manion, the groom's best man. In December 1933, they were married. Ten months later, my sister, Carole, was born, but the doctor said there had been problems in the delivery and it was unlikely she would have more children. My folks were fine with that and went on their merry way with their little daughter – for nine years – and then, much to their surprise, along came Susan – and then Virginia – and then me.

In the early years of their marriage, Dad worked at a bank briefly until he was hired at Kodak. He stayed there until his retirement in 1971. Mom worked at Sears. She also took art courses at Rochester Institute of Technology. She was a magnificent seamstress making many of her own clothes as well as ours. In a different day and age, she probably could have been an excellent dress designer. Her wardrobe was remarkable. She always dressed with class. I don't think she owned a pair of slacks till she was in her 40's or 50's – and then her slacks were typically white, yellow or gray. I have a photo of her in a rustic mountain setting on vacation wearing high heels, a dress and fur stole. She never wore flat shoes until she was in her 60's and then only to do yard work. She'd complain that she felt like she was walking in a hole in the ground. People marveled at how elegant she always looked.

She was nearly fanatical about neatness and orderliness. Our house was always spotless, everything in its place. I loved that about her. I loved coming home in the evening to find clean sheets and a turned-down bed. Table tops nor counters were ever sticky; never a crumb on the floor. She always put the couch or other furniture in front of the living room window. Couldn't risk finger prints, you know.

It was rare, when Dad wasn't home, to see her sitting down. She cleaned the whole basement regularly, washed down the walls of the house two or three times a year, painted every year or two, mowed, raked, shoveled snow, and cleaned and cleaned and cleaned. One of my funniest memories was during one of her wall-washing projects. Virginia and I were helping her move all the furniture. At one point, as I was sitting on a footstool in the middle of the living room, Mom took a sunburst clock off the wall, handed it to me and turned back to remove the sconces. The clock was huge and was poking my arms as I tried to hold it, and I said, "Prickly old bat!" Well, Mom swung around and swatted me right off the footstool. In an instant we realized Mom thought I was referring to her, and Virginia and I howled with laughter till we could hardly breathe. Needless to say, this became our new nickname for her. (Well, one of our nicknames – the other was "old paint.")

The other thing about the incident that made it so ridiculous was that Mom never hit any of us that I recall. When we were little, we were always sure she would. She would threaten us with a yardstick and even make us go get the thing out of the closet when we had done something wrong. In those days, parents had 'authority.' They didn't have to yell, or scream, or repeat, or hit. All they had to do was say, "Go get the stick!" and the errant child would collapse in a heap of apologies, swearing never to commit this particular offense again.

Mom was never so happy as when Dad was around. All the years he was at Kodak, he worked trick-work, but no matter what shift he was on, days, evenings or nights, she was always waiting for him. Sometimes she'd go meet him after work at his bowling league or at a bar. Other times, she'd have a meal waiting for him at home. They took vacations alone every year, often to the Adirondack Mountains or Canada. We girls would go someplace else. It seemed pretty normal. It never occurred to me that it was unusual for families not to vacation together.

About a year or so after Dad retired, they moved to Roswell, New Mexico. (It was an extremely small town and we'd tease them about having their '5:00 hurry minute' as opposed to a rush hour). They had had enough of the snow and cold. We would go out to visit every couple of years, but they never came back this way. They seemed to love it there, made lots of friends, traveled around the southwest. Mom adapted to small town living very quickly and became amazed by bigger cities. She wrote on 6/18/74: "They have a beautiful mall in Lubbock that makes Sibley's look like a has been. It even has a Tiffany jewelry store. I had the nerve to go in and ask if they had a peace ring – novelty jewelry no less. They were very polite when they said no and treated me as if I were just another eccentric."

In 1975, when they took their first plane ride. Note a couple things she had written before and after that occasion.

11/24/74: "We finally got to on the Boeing 747 I wrote you about before. I thoroughly enjoyed it. Three of them are being stored at the airport until the energy crisis is considered over. For you who have flown, it is probably old hat, but for us who have never been on a plane, it was quite an experience just standing still. Hard to believe the wingspan is wider than from the front curb to the back of our lot."

11/24/75: "Flying is out of this world! We love it – smooth as glass – if the weather is bad, we may change our minds though."

As time went on, Dad had more and more health problems and in the summer of 1986, Mom called to say he wasn't doing well. I took this to mean he was very, very sick, because they rarely told us when anything was wrong. 'Mustn't upset the girls.' In fact, a few years before, Dad called me on the phone one day – which he never did – to say that Mom had undergone a radical mastectomy that morning, but not to worry because she was fine. Surprise!

She did write about needing a hysterectomy on 4/25/73: "I'll be going into Eastern NM Medical Center on May 7 to be operated on May 8 – good old "Hysterectomy." Had a thorough biopsy a week ago and absolutely no cancer but could go into it so taking no chances. The street address is _____ just so you don't go wasting your money calling your Dad." Here's another instance where she decided to share with me one of Dad's issues. 5/4/77: "Your Dad had trouble just driving to the bank yesterday. He didn't tell me how he didn't want to go until he got home. He said he just can't judge distance any more and his eyes are getting worse. He has even gone so far as to suggest I do the driving now – unheard of before. Don't pass this on; your Dad prefers to wait until he is given a thorough examination. I won't tell Virginia why we won't go over just now, but will later on. That goes for the Aunts too. You know how he feels about getting people stirred up when there is nothing to tell."

As you can see, even then, she had qualifications.

So the fact that she called to say Dad wasn't well, was a major change on her part. I flew out there, got him in the hospital, and we discovered he had lung cancer. After they got him built up a bit and started radiation treatments, he was able to go back home and he did pretty well for several months. But in the spring of 1987, he started losing ground again and died the end of May.

During the various visits that my sisters and I made out to New Mexico during those months and on through the funeral, we noticed Mom was acting a bit oddly. For instance, when we were all in New Mexico for Dad's funeral, we were going to go out one afternoon. My sister, Susan, had some insurance papers that she was going through laid out on a table. We had a hard time convincing Mom to come along with us because she was sure someone would break into the house and steal the papers. We assured her they were of no value to anyone, but she wouldn't leave. Finally, she covered them with a dish towel. We laughed, thinking she was kidding, but she wasn't. Once the papers were covered, she was satisfied that they were safe and she came along quite willingly.

We wrote it off to the stress and grief of caring for and losing my Dad, but as time went on and she came to visit me or went to Arizona or Virginia to see my sisters, we came to the conclusion that this was not going away. In fact, it was becoming more troublesome. On one visit in Arizona, Carole wasn't feeling well. Normally, Mom would have been solicitous, but not hovering. Well, in this instance, she felt the need to sit by Carole's bedside and stroke her arm … and stroke her arm … and stroke … and rub … and rub, etc. etc. until the hair on her arm formed little balls. Carole's housemate, Jude, tried her utmost to distract Mom, but to no avail.

We also got some reports from her friends and neighbors in Roswell that she wasn't herself. Concern was increasing all around.

One of Mom's friends told us of a picnic they attended. Mom had brought a salad to the picnic and, later in the day, when her friends were ready to drive her home, she wanted her bowl back. The leftover salad was sitting in the middle of the table and the hosts were busy with other guests, so Mom's friend suggested she leave it and pick it up the next day. Typically, Mom would have agreed, or at most, put the salad in another container and washed out her own bowl. But in this instance, totally out of character, she got highly agitated at the prospect of losing her bowl and proceeded to dump the salad onto the table and walk away with the dirty bowl.

One day, Mom called to tell me that "a very nice policeman" followed her home and told her she had to come to the police station the next day and apologize for what she had done. I never did ascertain what, in fact, actually happened, but my guess was that she had broken some traffic law, the policeman followed her to insure that she got home safely, and she had to pay a ticket the next day. Fortunately, she lived in a very small town where people knew her and looked out for her up to the time we finally got her to move back east.

Mom was a prolific letter writer and as I was going back and reading the hundreds of letters she wrote me from 1972 through 1988, it became obvious that there was a change in her writing ability the last year or so. At the time, I didn't really see the pattern. Note that at this time, she starts referring to my Dad as George, something she had never done in my letters. And notice the kind of vague, run-on sentences. 4/6/87: "I had hopes of getting at least a note out to you right after George's eye test and medical examination. While he (George) was waiting for the dilation to clear, he took me – my appointment was the cataract checkup – that didn't take long it wasn't ready he said. However, when George was in another room, the doctor- said the growth was slow but if necessary, any sooner, than expected go back but he advised about another year." And this one from 1/17/88: "This will be later than I said. The holiday got in the way. The Post Office also took the holiday no mail going out or in. I am on the way today though right now, the celebration lasted over the weekend and also on Monday." (She signed it "Mom" Mother)

I've often thought that one of the saddest things about Mom getting Alzheimer's was that, in spite of her close relationship with our Dad, she was also quite independent and optimistic. I think she would have had an active and full life even after he was gone. As you will see in the letters over the next 12 years, she had no other physical health problems.

Her letters to me were, for the most part, surface topics, nothing personal or revealing of how she felt about anything. Less than a month after

Dad died, I got a letter about visitors she had had, insurance papers and whom she had sent thank you cards to. But look what she wrote to Aunt Mary and Aunt Anne on the same day:

"This most devoted wife is falling by the wayside, I think I am falling apart. I come out of the living room or any other room for that matter and say: "How about if we have supper early tonight," and stop short of looking at his chair – empty. I catch myself doing that a lot. I believe I have a cure though.

"My dear friend and neighbor went to the hospital nearly every day – the times he was home she would come over and visit us just for a while to break the monotony and those times brightened the day for both of us. Sad to say, her husband was buried yesterday. He had been in the hospital just ten days. Through the days of George's death and burial, Doris baked and cooked and went out of her way to keep things going – so – I had to (wanted to) repay in kind, right? Well, I sure did – cooked, shopped, drove, the whole bit, and as of now I feel great – I can't stand a crybaby – I do it some, but I can't stand it.

"Doris called this afternoon and asked me to go over. I did and was there for a while when Doris got weepy. I thought I had better come home, but changed my mind and thought crying won't help anything; if you feel it coming on say a prayer instead. Hope it works."

* * * * * *

In the spring of 1989, I had Mom come back east for a visit. We were going to have her stay with Aunt Mary and try to determine if she could manage on her own if she moved back to Rochester. It was during that visit that I fully realized what we were up against. She didn't recall ever having been at my house before. She had trouble writing checks or making change. She had this rather vague, but pleasant way of greeting people, not knowing whether it was someone she was supposed to know. These weren't isolated incidents caused by grief. She was clearly regressing and the incidents were getting more and more frequent. We had been encouraging her to move from New Mexico to either Arizona where my sisters lived, or back east to New York, but she wouldn't agree, mainly because Dad was buried in Roswell.

However, that spring time visit caused us to insist she move, and fortunately, she finally did agree.

I think part of the reason she agreed was because she had begun to worry about so many things and seem to recognize that she couldn't keep things straight on her own. Note this letter from 4/88 written a month before Virginia's son, Daniel was born: "I think I'm going to be in trouble. Virginia called last week and said, "Well, what is it?" I said, what did you get? We kidded around a bit about twins etc., and that was it. Just now it came to me she must have been trying to find out when I would go over to their house to be with the children. She mentioned Mike coming over here and it never struck me she said they would have the use of an apartment if Doris wanted to come so the children wouldn't give up their rooms because they were used to them. It never occurred to me. I called right then and there but Bill and Virginia were out. Jessica answered so I told her to have them call when they got home. Time went by and I thought Jessica may have forgotten so I called again, not home yet! The next morning I called Bill at work and he said he would straighten it out with her, Mike would be going to their house to help Bill put on new tile in the kitchen and Mike would be coming over here when he got out of school to take me back to their place after the baby is born. Glad I called, so I could stop worrying – two worries with just one stop!"

During this 1987-89 time-frame, Susan was handling the insurance and business issues surrounding Dad's death. Carole and Virginia were keeping tabs on Mom as best they could and eventually took care of selling the house and its contents and packing up the things we would keep as well as the items Mom wanted to bring with her.

In August, my husband, Gary, went to bring Mom back to live with us. She waited eagerly for him to come. She called on the phone frequently to reassure herself that Gary would take care of everything. But after he went out there, helped her close her bank accounts, pay off final bills and pack, she was convinced he had stolen all her money. She would barely speak to him by the time they got back here and I had to tell her over and over that the checks she brought were, indeed, all her money. Once we opened her bank account here, it was easier for her to understand because she could see the actual numbers written in the bank book. However, it set a precedent for her that left Gary in a suspicious light ever after.

We had a bedroom/bath addition built on the house for her, and we all generally felt better about having Mom in a safe place where she wouldn't be alone. There was a notable deterioration in Mom's condition shortly after she moved in with us. It was as if she suddenly realized that she no longer had to struggle by herself to keep things together – that Gary and I would remember the important things for her.

That Christmas, we bought our first computer and the convenience of it led me to write a series of letters to my sisters on the day to day activities here living with Alzheimer's. (I eventually added a couple of my aunts to the mailing list as well). These letters tell Mom's story and mine, as we wandered through two years of fascinating and devastating changes. Then there were intermittent letters when Mom moved to a nursing home and more frequent letters again surrounding her final days and her death.

At the time these letters began, my husband, Gary, was teaching at Monroe Community College, our son David was a student at Rochester Institute of Technology and was living at home, and our daughter Michelle was a student at Boston College. My sisters, Carole and Virginia lived in Phoenix, and Susan lived in Virginia Beach. Susan subsequently moved to Phoenix in 1992.

CHAPTER 2

In which we learn the ground rules – there aren't any.

January 2, 1990

    I've been playing with our new computer the past few days and I suppose it's time I started writing a real letter. Actually, I probably wouldn't be doing this if it weren't for our new toy. I sat down to experiment with it the other day and realized I can type all this in and print out copies for the three of you. If I waited for the ambition to hand-write three letters . . . well, maybe some time before 1999.

    As you all know, I took Mom to a Geriatric Assessment Center just before Thanksgiving. They did a very thorough job; physical, mental, nutritional and social assessments. They did x-rays, special geriatric blood work, neurological exam, EKG, and I don't remember what else. The point is, they said if there were any contributing factors to her dementia, they would find them. We also lined her up with a personal physician, a woman doctor who did her residency at the Assessment Center. After the initial visit (three and a half hours), they called and said they wanted her to go for an MRI scan (magnetic resonance imaging) and a neuropsychiatric exam. Well, I had to do a song and dance to get her to the MRI appointment. She didn't want any part of it. Then afterwards she said, "Well, that was easy!"

January 11, 1990

    I seem to be having trouble sticking to this don't I? Well, the last time I was here, Michelle came in and wanted me to go into Prodigy to find out the weather in Pennsylvania since she was going there the next day, and I haven't been able to get back to this till now.

As far as the neuropsych exam, I called the doctor (a psychologist) who would be doing it and I asked a bunch of pesky questions. Bottom line was, it would be a 3 to 4 hour test including things like putting blocks into holes, eye:hand coordination, pencil and paper type tests and short-term memory. The point of all this was to see what her level of skill is so they could advise me better on how to deal with her. Phooey! I know perfectly well what her level of skill is.

The only person I dealt with at the center who made me uncomfortable was a sociologist or a social worker. I'm not sure exactly what she was, but she certainly didn't seem to recognize that a family member might know what they're talking about. On the one hand, she said things like, "You can't treat her like a child. She has to feel independent as long as possible." Then she turned around and told me I should get her into an adult day care program whether she liked it or not. I told this woman that when day care was appropriate, I would know, and this certainly wasn't the time. She insisted this certainly was the time and that Mom needed socialization with her peers. Oh, right! A woman who never joined a club or organization in her life, who never had coffee with neighbors, who was seemingly happy in her own home, and now is quite happy in mine and who has just gotten over the idea that I was going to ship her off to a nursing home when she wasn't looking! This person needs to be carted off to a day care center every day to try to socialize with a group of people who are, at least at the moment, further down the road of Alzheimer's than she is. The sociologist assured me that even if she protests, it means she's using her brain to do that and socialization would reduce her stress. That's what she thinks. Right now Mom doesn't get too stressed out very often, but if we put her in day care, she sure as heck would.

Anyway, when I went back to the Assessment Center[1], the doctor said, "The good news is that there's nothing physically wrong with your mother. The bad news is, there's nothing physically wrong with your mother." That about said it. They could find no contributing factors. The blood work and everything else was quite normal. While they can't positively diagnose Alzheimer's, they eliminated everything else. It's pretty much what I expected. They're going to send me copies of the reports. I was waiting for them so I could send copies to you, but they haven't come yet, so I decided to get this letter out anyway.

Day to day, we do pretty well. Gary hasn't gotten the knack of going with the flow, at least not all the time. He often thinks if he just hollers at her as he does with his mother, she'll respond appropriately. Guess what? She doesn't. But I think she's getting used to him. She's a little less paranoid about him than she used to be, but if push comes to shove, and something is wrong, she assumes he's to blame somehow.

Before Thanksgiving, all she talked about was going to see Susan, etc. for the holiday. She'd ask me every little while if we were really going, could she come too, and when would we leave, and how long would we stay, etc. At it turns out, the change of pace, the long drive there and back, all the people, and of course, two dogs, all took their toll. The week before we went, David took the train to Boston to spend time with Michelle, and then they met us at Jacqui & Michael's.[2]

Up until that time, I had a feeling that Mom didn't know who Michelle was. There was never a sign of recognition when we mentioned her name. When we got to Jacqui's, Mom greeted Michelle warmly. So I thought that she knew her on sight. All while we were there, Mom spent just about every moment cleaning and tidying, cleaning and tidying, cleaning and tidying. At about the point when Susan had had enough, she asked, "Do you really think that if you weren't here, none of this work would get done?!" Mom's response was, "Of course it wouldn't."

We took Michelle back to the train station the day before we left for home and Mom never commented. But then, on our way home, she started telling David that when we got home, there was a bedroom for Gary and me, and one for her, and another one where he and his wife could stay when they came to visit. David said he wasn't married, but she ignored that. Then she couldn't figure out why he was with us and not with Michelle. By the time we got home, she was wandering around trying to figure out where everyone was going to sleep. She decided she could put up a divider in her room so David could sleep there, and then he could sleep in the upstairs room when his wife got here. David (who <u>does</u> have the knack of going with the flow) said, "Supposing I just sleep in David's room?" She asked where that was and he pointed it out. She thought this was a fine solution, but that he could only stay for a couple of days. He tried to tell her again that he wasn't married, but she didn't believe him. So I brilliantly said, "He's not married! He only lives with that girl!" That didn't go over too well, so I explained how Michelle was his sister, my daughter, and she slept in her own room when she was home from college, and that she'd be coming home for Christmas. To which she responded, "Not unless he marries her, she won't!" We gave up. After a couple of days, she came back down to earth and realized that David belonged here.

Now Michelle is home, but I'm not at all sure Mom knows who she is. The first two weeks she kept calling her 'that girl.' Now she knows her name and has a pretty good idea that she's related to me, but that's as far as it goes. Oh well . . . maybe when she's here longer in the summer.

The only real snag we've hit so far that I haven't found a solution for (there have been a lot of snags, but we've resolved them to one degree or another) is when the kids have their friends over. They're only here about an hour when Mom starts telling David or Michelle that these people really should go home. After a bit, she starts dropping broad hints directly to their friends. The kids were going to have a New Year's Eve party while we were in Nashville and I told Mom that David was in charge, but luckily, the party was moved to someone else's house so it didn't become a problem. They did, however, have a gathering the night we came home. I spent half the evening trying to keep Mom away from the kids. Gary and I usually visit for a few minutes and then go upstairs to watch TV. We told Mom to go in her room and ignore the kids, but no dice. She plunked herself down in the living room and tried to join in. Then she started telling them to go home. Michelle came up for help and Mom was right on her heels. Gary told her again to leave the kids alone and either stay with us or go to her own room. She wouldn't agree to either. Finally about 10:30 p.m., I went down to tell her that 'Newhart' was on TV and she should watch it. The kids were watching football. No way. So I said I'd go watch it by myself in her room. She followed me in and sat down to watch with me, but every two minutes she'd jump up and think of another excuse to go back out. "Those two on the couch shouldn't be drinking." "They're drinking pop, Mom." "Well, they'll get all popped out. I'd better go tell them." "Sit down and stay here." "Maybe I should go tell them Newhart's on." "Sit down and stay put." "I think those two on the couch are bored with football. Let's invite them in here." "Sit down! And leave them alone!" Just about the time Newhart ended, David called, "Pizza's here!" Mom jumped up again and ran out saying "He said we can come out now!" So I let her have some pizza and coke. Then I told her it was late and to go to bed. Now she decides to clean up. The kids had three pizzas and multiple cokes all over the living room floor. She kept going out, standing in front of the TV and taking stock. We kept telling her to leave things alone, the kids weren't through eating, that's John's coke, leave it alone, David will get that, get away from the TV etc. etc. etc. Finally, I had to out and out holler at her. I was standing in the kitchen door and told her to leave everything alone and go to her room, NOW!!! And I pointed. She said, "All right, but I'm going this way," and she made her exit through the dining room. I told the kids to let me know if she reappeared, but she didn't.

As I said, I'm not sure yet what to do about this one. The kids are great and try to understand, but this whole business has got to be making them uncomfortable. The next thing you know, they won't come by any more. I'd hate for David and Michelle to reach a point where they don't feel they can invite anyone over any more. It's happened three times so far. We've told her we like these kids, it's David and Michelle's house too, and they can stay as late as they want to, but it doesn't help. We'll think of something. Maybe handcuffs . . . nah!

Financially, things are on an even keel for her. We have transferred all her accounts to Citibank, the bulk of it in a money market and the rest in checking. She long ago gave up the idea that Gary had stolen her money, but she really doesn't understand the bank either. Some days she wants every cent she has to be deposited in the bank. Other days she wants it all out so she can see it. And yet other days she thinks she has no money whatsoever. She easily agreed to let me put my name on the account, so we're covered in case I need to pay bills (day-care, home-aide, etc.) when she really gets out in left field.

She knows she has four daughters, but she doesn't always know who I'm talking about when I mention you by name. Sometimes she does. She particularly remembers Susan since she's seen her most recently, and I suppose I talk about Susan more because we see each other fairly often. The grandchildren are a blur, but if I show her pictures, she knows who they are. It's curious. She can pluck information out of the distant past far more easily than the recent past. I guess that's a common trait. Aunt Therese used to tell me stories about when she was a girl as if it were last week and at the same time, she couldn't think how to get in or out of the car.

Speaking of Aunts, I miss Aunt Mary! It's strange going through her apartment, sorting through her things. Jerry and Marcy[3] and I go over once or twice a week and make a dent, but we can only work for just so long before one of us gets depressed and we all go home. We're almost done getting rid of junk, giving away clothes, and so on. They really had little of value. Some of the furniture, Jerry and Marcy kept. There was nothing I really wanted because I have nowhere to put excess furniture, but we did bring her TV for Mom. Whatever is left – dishes, appliances, books – we're going to sell at a household sale right there at the apartment. That way, we don't have to move anything out.

We haven't told Aunt Anne, but we think she has a sense of it anyway. Jerry told her Aunt Mary was sick and wouldn't be able to come back for a long time. She doesn't mention her name, but seems to cry a lot more than she used to and you can't always tell why. She doesn't speak plainly, just makes sounds or rambles, but now and then you can pick out a word or two that might give you a hint of what she's trying to say. She says the word 'scared' oftentimes when she cries. That's sad because you don't know how to help.

Well, on to brighter topics. I don't know any. Wait, how's this? It's been fun having Michelle home for the holidays. My boss is going to Indonesia on business and – eeks – I have to play supervisor for 2 ½ weeks. Gary's being lazy. Nobody should be allowed to have so much vacation time when his wife has to work. The decent spouse would at least get up at 5:30 a.m., go out in the cold and pretend he has somewhere to go.

Well, I better quit while I'm ahead. I may write more often now that I have this nifty word processor. Susan, Gary had trouble with his camera, so all the Thanksgiving pictures didn't come out, but the ones that did are quite good.

P.S. Did you know that in 1 Samuel 7:12, Samuel finds a stone and names it Ebenezer? Weird, those Bible folk.

[1]*When it came time to go back for the results of her tests, Mom refused to go. When I got home from the appointment, she absolutely did not want to hear about it. Even though we didn't mention the word 'Alzheimer's,' I think she knew full well what we were looking for and didn't want to face it.*

[2]*Jacqui & Michael are Susan's daughter and son-in-law. We were having our Thanksgiving holiday at their home in Maryland and Susan was coming up from Virginia.*

[3]*Jerry and Marcy are my cousin and his wife. Among the three of us, we pretty much looked out for the 3 aunts. Aunt Mary died of a heart attack in November 1989. Mom went with me to the funeral home but kept asking when we were going to see my friend and "Who is that man lying over there?"*

January 16, 1990

Well, here we go again. I guess I'll just keep a running commentary of what's going on here so you might feel like you're a little closer to the action or something.

The odd things Mom says or does can usually be tied back to something that's been said or done around her recently, but just when you think you're getting used to the status quo, she comes up with something new and I'm taken by surprise. Today when I came home from work, she told me that last night, when I wasn't here, she saw some sort of pink lights in the stairway and then a face on the wall that moved over the clock, grinned at her and disappeared. She said she thought that someone upstairs was playing with a camera or something, but when she looked up the stairs, no one was there. It sounds eerie, but it didn't sound as if it frightened her. She was just kind of curious about it. I haven't had a chance to ask Gary or David about this so I'm not sure if there's any explanation to it. It may just be something she dreamed, or (I hope not) she may have started hallucinating. Aunt Anne started doing that real early in the game. There were always people upstairs or downstairs, getting in her way or making so much noise she couldn't sleep, or sleeping in her bed. Once she told us St. Anne and St. Joachim were in the back hallway (the coats hanging on the wall). Fortunately, she didn't seem afraid of these people at all, just annoyed with them for the most part. The people in her bed were taking up too much room and the saints in the hallway wouldn't come in.

I mentioned a few days ago that we went to Nashville for New Year's. We wouldn't have gone if David and Michelle hadn't been here. When Mom first moved here, I thought since she managed – more or less – on her own in New Mexico that an occasional weekend alone here wouldn't be a problem. In October, we went to Boston and before we left, I gave Mom the garage door opener because we were expecting a delivery of plumbing parts for the addition. Well, apparently, Saturday night, she started playing with it. She'd push the button over and over and when she'd stop, the door would be partially or fully open. So about 10:00 pm, she went next door and asked for help. Our neighbor came over, closed the door and sent her inside. But not being one to leave well enough alone, Mom went back out a while later and did it again. This time she got our neighbor out of bed. By the third go around, he came over, closed the door, sent her inside and kept the garage door opener.

In November, we went to New York City to meet Susan and Charlie. This time, we got home Sunday evening to find a note on the door from the neighbor on the other side saying Mom was at their house sleeping. She had locked herself out and we could come get her the next morning. So much for leaving her alone weekends . . .

CHAPTER 3

In which we adjust to there being no ground rules.

January 22, 1990

Not much new to report. Michelle has gone back to school. We think Mom had a pretty good idea who she was before she left. For the moment, she knows Michelle will be back in the summer. However, she is not at all thrilled with how messy 'that girl' is. She asked me periodically while Michelle was home if I didn't think her room was just horrible. The implication was that I should get busy and clean it, or have Michelle clean it, or (hope, hope) maybe I'd let her clean it. I was no help. I'd just say something noncommittal like, "Yeah, it's horrible. Don't look at it."

I turned off the phones the other night because we were going to be out and we never get messages – or at least we never get them straight – when people call. Friday, David came home to hear this long speech about three phone calls which, the best he could figure out were Michelle and two other people, one probably a salesman. He thought they all indicated that they would call back. So when we were all going to be out that evening, I saw no point in putting Mom through more phone calls she couldn't decipher, so I turned the phones off. Later, Gary got the long explanation about the three previous calls and surmised it was Virginia and two other people, one probably a salesman. Who knows. So unless we're home, we're never sure if any of you have called. We talked to Michelle the next day and she said that she had called in the evening and assumed we were all out because no one answered. So it wasn't her during the day. So "Hi, Virginia. Nice of you to call … I think …"

January 24, 1990

Virginia, a bit of trivia for you guys, especially Michael. You know those Colonel's insignias we sent from Gary's Dad? Well, Gary just found out that there are two types of eagles. The eagle holds arrows in his right foot and an olive branch in his left foot. If the eagle's head is facing the branch, the insignia was issued during peace time or at least out of any war zone. If the eagle is facing the arrows, the insignia was issued during the war. Gen. MacArthur had those 'war eagles' especially made during World War II and then stopped making them. So now they're collectors' items and rather valuable. I think I sent Mike one of each but I'm not sure. We found three eagles here, two 'war eagles' and a regular one which David had. (Now David has one of each). So have Mike check. Interesting, huh?[1]

I keep realizing over and over again that Mom is a lot like the kids when they were little. I have to act accordingly. I told her a few days ago that we were going to go to a color guard show on Saturday, thinking it would give her something to look forward to. Well, it did, but ever since, she asks me every day when we're going and where we're going and what she should wear, etc. This is the type of thing I tried to avoid with David and Michelle when they were small. I'd never tell them of an upcoming event until it was upon us so they wouldn't bug me for days; besides which, they had little concept of time.

I find myself thinking things like, "She should learn to ignore sales pitches on the phone or in the mail." She thinks she has to respond to or buy everything she gets ads for. But then I remind myself that she's 'unlearning' as she goes along.

The picture thing hasn't exactly gone away.[2] She's got the idea that I don't approve and so now she rarely does it in front of me. Initially, she'd bring out the pictures or make a production of talking to them almost as if she was showing off. When I ignored her or expressed disapproval, she finally stopped. Now, every once in a while, she'll make some comment about what she said to one of them earlier and how they responded. I told her the other day that they're just pictures and they don't respond, but she said she likes to talk to them anyway. David says she does it quite often when I'm not around.

Yesterday she finished reading the book by Bill Cosby, "Fatherhood." When she brought it upstairs to put it away, David and I happened to be watching Cosby on TV. She got all excited and said, "There he is! The one who's been smiling at me all week." She held the book up to the TV so the picture on the cover could 'see himself' on TV. She started telling the picture on the book, "See, there you are, and there's your wife. Now look right there." I told her she was making it very difficult to see the television as she was right in front of it. So then she squatted down on the floor with the book and just stayed there with it for about 15 minutes. Every little while she'd comment about how Cosby (on TV) wouldn't look her way and see himself. Finally when a commercial came on, she put the book away and went back downstairs.

Am I boring you with all this Mom stuff? If so, you can just dispose of my letters when they show up if you like. It's just that these little occurrences are such a large part of my day-to-day life, it doesn't seem like much else new is happening. And, too, I thought it would give you a chance to kind of track her progress (?) if you are so inclined. When you've had enough, just holler. Actually, to a large extent, I find this somewhat fascinating; to observe first-hand the changes in a person's mind.

Let's see, what else is new? My boss has been away for two weeks and I've been in charge. It's fun for a while but I'll be glad when he's back. I was sure I'd get a lot done since he wouldn't be around to give me work every little while, but it turns out his boss has filled in the void quite nicely.

Gary has finally gone back to work. I use the term 'work' rather loosely here. After a month off for Christmas, he goes back to a really rugged schedule. Mon., Wed. and Fri. he has classes from 8:00 a.m. to noon. Tues. and Thurs., he has classes from 8:00 a.m. till 1:00 p.m. I think I'll kill him in his sleep one day. I know I'm in the wrong business. He makes more money than I do too. Grrr!

[1]*Virginia's husband, Bill, is Gary's brother. Michael is their oldest son. When Gary & Bill's Dad, a retired Army General, died in September 1988, we distributed much of his military paraphernalia to the grandchildren.*

[2]*The picture thing was a bizarre occurrence that started when Mom was still in New Mexico. She had pictures of Dad, the Pope and Christ that she called 'her boys.' She'd talk to them, line them up in front of the TV for 'their favorite shows,' have them watch for the mailman for her, etc. It was truly weird.*

March 25, 1990

Gary took off for New York this morning. He'll be back Wednesday night. Oh boy, four days of spending quality time with Mom. Whenever I start to talk to her, I get the instant response of "Huh?" When she does hear me, most of the time she doesn't understand me – and I get annoyed. So if I don't talk to her to avoid getting (unjustifiably) annoyed, she thinks I'm mad or sick and she hovers. There's got to be a happy medium.

She managed to lose almost $200 this weekend. She wanted cash, so on Friday after work, I took her to the bank and got her $200. She counted it and put it in her wallet. We went directly from there to Wegman's and she bought about $12 worth of groceries. I watched her put $8 change back in her wallet and we went home. None of us went out that evening. Saturday morning I took her to church, we came home and never went out again during the day. Gary and I were going out to dinner with friends that evening so Gary gave David $10 to get himself and Mom some food. I told Mom that David was going to church and then he'd bring her something to eat. He left and shortly thereafter, we left. Mom was not a happy camper. (Susan, she really did a Mandy routine over being left alone).[3]

When we got home last night about 10:00 p.m., she was dozing in a chair. Gary went up to pack and a few minutes later came down and woke her up to iron a shirt for him. After a good 15 minutes of disorientation, she finally realized what she was doing and ironed the shirt. After that she sat down and started telling me this long story about David. Somehow, wading through this very difficult discourse, I concluded that David brought in this large box – he kept going outside to talk to his friends, but they wouldn't come in – she couldn't get him to tell her how he paid for the food – she didn't want him and his friends to pay because they don't work – the mothers and fathers should be paying – he gave her half the food and they all had the other half – and I should straighten out this whole mess.

Today I got David's story. He came home from church, called to have pizza delivered, the guy delivered it, David paid for it, he and Mom ate and later, he got in his car and went out. His friends were never here at all.

The point of this little digression into David's adventures is that she discovered the money was missing during the evening and is now convinced that 'his friends,' who were supposedly outside had something to do with it. We tried all afternoon to convince her that no one was here and that the pizza man never came in the house, and that David paid for the pizza with Gary's money. Which, of course, put her on to another suspect. Where do you suppose Gary got the money, hhhmmmmm? After a while she finally admitted that she really didn't think that David or Gary would take her money, but maybe – just maybe – Gary accidentally got the money in his suitcase before he went out the door this morning.

I finally went out in the kitchen to make brownies and the money was forgotten for the moment. Later, I filled out all her tax forms and had her sign them. (She will pay no federal taxes, but I had to file because of the house sale. She'll take the once-in-a-lifetime exclusion. I didn't intend to file New Mexico state taxes, but Doris sent me forms that included one which might get her a $250 refund on property taxes. I'm not sure because one form said she had to be living in NM on the last day of the year AND have lived there at least six months, and the other form said she had to be living there on the last day OR have lived there at least six months. So I sent it in; we'll see). Anyway, I had her sign all the appropriate forms and told her about the possible refund. And what did she ask? "Do you suppose this refund has anything to do with my money that's missing?" I never learn. David later said I missed my cue. If I were sure she was going to get it, I should have said yes, NM took your money and they're sorry so they're sending you an extra $50 to make up for it.

[3]*Mandy is Susan's dog and a truly unique personality.*

April 2, 1990

Well, the money never turned up. Heaven knows what happened. The only thing I can think of is that when we went to the grocery store after the bank, she took the money out and laid it on the counter (she has a habit of putting money on the conveyor belt in the store – lost a whole bunch of change one day doing that) and then turned away to pay for her items and bingo! someone stole it. Either that, or one day, way down the road, the money is going to turn up somewhere in this house when we least expect it.

April 6, 1990

Well, I took Mom to the bank today and got her another $200. We'll see how long this one lasts. As we were on our way out the door, Gary said, "DON'T stop at the store!" We didn't.

I went to a Caregivers Seminar last night. It was put on by the Alzheimer's Disease and Related Disorders Association. They sponsor seminars like this one, support groups, research, etc. I found a support group nearby and I've been to a few meetings. About 10 or 12 people come to this one. Most of them are older people caring for their spouses or people with a relative in a nursing home. No one else is caring for a parent.

I have a friend who recently got a job as volunteer coordinator for a group that provides occasional respite for Alzheimer's families. She was at the last support group meeting I went to and the other people there seemed to be pleased she was there, but she wasn't given a chance to say much. Anyone who had questions had to wait till after the meeting to talk to her. Every meeting is about the same. Everyone tells whom he or she is caring for and a bit about their background. Once you've been to two or three meetings, it gets a bit repetitious.

Anyway, the seminar last night was excellent. There were speakers from nursing homes, day-care centers, people from the ADRDA, a doctor, an occupational therapist and a recreational therapist. They had a lot of good information and a really useful video on caring for Alzheimer's patients at home. There was a ton of literature and a panel for answering questions during the last half-hour. They have these types of seminars every couple of months. Could be really helpful as time goes on.

April 9, 1990

Well, Mom gave us a new little challenge last night. I had gone to bed about 9:30 p.m. and I thought she had too, but David told me later that she went in her room for about ten minutes and came back out. She fell asleep watching TV. He and Gary didn't pay any attention. About 11:00 p.m. I woke up to hear Gary say, "Hey! Where are you going?" Mom said, "Out." He didn't respond or move because he didn't think she would really go anywhere, but then she opened the front door, went out and pulled the door shut behind her. Gary jumped up and opened the front door and said, "Where are you going?! Get back in here!" She came right in and he told her to go to bed. She said she wasn't going to because I wasn't in bed, but he assured her I had been in bed a long time. So she started up the stairs and he had to redirect her to her own room. Needless to say, I slept with one ear open the rest of the night.

By the way, Carole, I got the box of letters you sent. But did you have to send them in a frozen vegetable box? They were in the freezer when I got home. Mom took them out to show me, but I had a hard time convincing her to let me open the box to see what was inside. It said 'Keep frozen' and that was that. She did have a fun time going through them once she discovered what it was though, especially looking at the letters David and Michelle sent her when they were little. (I might add, Michelle and David also had a good time over those).

Aunt Nan is back from California.[4] YAY!!! She came over to see Mom today and it really made Mom's day.

---

[4] *Aunt Nan is Mom's sister-in-law and lifelong friend. Her husband, Mom's brother Kernan, had died some years before. Aunt Nan lived in Rochester while Mom was with me, but now lives in California with her daughter.*

CHAPTER 4

More losses, surprises, frustrations

April 20, 1990

It's been a strange week – sort of the norm here, I guess.

Last Saturday a woman came over from ACCESS about a research program for Alzheimer's patients. It's a three-year program and the main purpose is to convince Medicare and other insurance companies that it's better to provide care in the home. People will keep their family member home longer and it will cost less over the long term. Participants will be assigned to the study group or the control group. The study group will be given $240/month to use for adult day care, in home aides or medical devices. Both groups are followed monthly by a caseworker.

I filled out an application and a nurse from ACCESS came for an interview. She was due at 1:00 p.m. so Gary took Mom out just before 1:00. I had been told the interview with me would take about an hour, and with Mom, about 15 minutes. The nurse asked all sorts of questions about Mom's current level of confusion and what sort of assistance I get, etc. We were almost finished when Gary and Mom came back. Then she started asking Mom questions to evaluate her condition. I was surprised how well Mom tolerated the questions because some of them were really simplistic, but Mom didn't seem to be bothered by it. She asked the day, date, where we live, the city and county. She asked Mom to take a piece of paper in her right hand, fold it, then put it on the floor. She had her read a sentence, write a sentence and draw a figure that was on a paper. (She did that REALLY well). Mom told her it was Saturday, March 17, 1978. She was able to do the physical stuff pretty well, but messed up on the information quite a bit. It took about 20 minutes, and Mom took it pretty well. You never know.

I found out today we're in the ACCESS control group. Oh well, somebody has to do it.

The day before yesterday, I was filling out some insurance forms so I could submit Mom's (and Aunt Mary's) medical bills to Blue Cross/Blue Shield. After I had them filled out, I asked her to sign the claim form. I explained that these were bills she had already paid (after Medicare did their part) and now we were submitting them to the other insurance company to see if they would pay their part. It never occurred to me that she'd get upset, but she hemmed and hawed and stewed and read every word on the claim form. I had to ask her several times to sign it. She said she didn't want to get herself into anything. I couldn't convince her that she wasn't paying anything, that this was to collect money. Then she asked if it was next month. I asked what 'it' was. She said, "This." She pointed to the insurance papers. I said it had to do with doctor appointments she had last November, but I knew I was losing ground. She was making less and less sense. She did finally sign it and I assured her everything was fine. A few minutes later she said, in a very annoyed manner, "Well, are you going to tell me?!" I said, "Tell you what?" and she said, "Whether or not it's next month." I finally discovered she was talking about an upcoming eye appointment, so I resolved that, but now she was upset and restless. She got up and started walking all around the house. I asked if she was looking for something. She said yes, the phone. I told her it was in the kitchen and she said, "Not that one! The other one!" I told her the other phone was upstairs, but she insisted there was another one downstairs. Finally she went upstairs and started looking around in our room, Michelle's room and opened David's door to look in his room till she found he was in there doing homework. He asked what she was looking for and she said the thing that goes under the phone. He took a couple of guesses to no avail. She came back down, wringing her hands, with David on her heels trying to help. Then she said it was right next to one of the chairs in the living room. There was nothing there, but she kept insisting and finally I got it. She was making a motion like she was opening a drawer and she said she had to make sure the papers were still there and okay. She was looking for her nightstand. I told her to go in her room and look next to her bed. She said, "Oh! I'm so confused!" But she went. She was in there for a while and came back out with four envelopes. She squirrels away letters, junk mail, receipts, etc. in her nightstand drawer. Every now and then, she'll pull a few out and carry them around with her all day or bring them to me to go over them and explain what they are and that they've been taken care of. Gary keeps telling her to throw the stuff away, but she gets even more frantic if you try to do that.

P.S. Tuesday night an attorney friend of Gary's came over and we had a Power of Attorney drawn up for me on behalf of Mom and for Gary on behalf of his Mom. Mrs. Thompson thought it was a good idea and agreed to come over the same night so Mom would see we weren't trying to pull the wool over her eyes.

April 28, 1990

Mom and I went to a wedding shower for Mark's fiance, Debbie, today.[5] It was interesting. She was delighted to be there and seemed to be enjoying the decorations and everything, but when she spotted all the gifts, she got really excited. Unfortunately, she assumed they were for her – or least some of them should be. When Debbie was opening them, I really felt badly because Mom would get all enthused as Nora picked up each one, and then she'd be really disappointed when she gave each one to Debbie. It was so sad. She was like a tiny child at another child's birthday party. Luckily, Nora (bless her) saved the day by making sure Mom got one of the prizes for the games. It was just a decorative kitchen towel, but Mom was happy as a clam to have a present to open.

[5]Nora and Mark are Gary's niece and nephew.

May 14, 1990

The reason I haven't written in a while is that we've been remodeling and redecorating our bedroom. I happened to mention around Easter time that I didn't have enough closet space and the next thing I knew, our room was full of sawdust and tools and I was sleeping in Michelle's room. I moved out of our room real early in the game. I told Gary he should too, but he wouldn't. I said everything was COVERED with dust, and he said he was too. I guess he had become one with his dust. But after a time, he had to take the bed apart and move everything to the center of the room so we could paint. Then I was sorry I encouraged him to move into Michelle's. When you've slept in a king-size bed for several years, going back to a double is like sleeping in a milkbox or something. Talk about crowded! Besides which, he always stays up late and when he'd come to bed, he had to wend his way through a tiny little path we had made from the door to Michelle's bed. Half our stuff was in her room. Gary tends to be a tad less than graceful on his best day. Imagine the racket he makes in the dark, climbing over furniture.

May 15, 1990

Before I forget to tell you, I recently read an article in our local paper on Alzheimer's and in the article was information about a doctor at UCLA who is doing a major research study on the children and siblings of Alzheimer's victims. Apparently he's gotten quite a bit of government funding and the participants in the study are getting free medical tracking over a period of time to see if a pattern or clue or predictor can be found. Just today I sent a letter to him to find out more about the study. The paper didn't indicate if this was a nation-wide study or just local to the Los Angeles area. But it did say he needs lots more people.

May 17, 1990

Here's a new turn of events in our household. I think I've told you I never know what's going to set Mom off or what she'll take in stride. Sometimes I'm so careful about the things I think will upset her, like when the social worker came for that interview and, as it turned out, it didn't seem to bother her in the least. For some months now, Mom's been complaining that she can't see well out of her right eye. A couple of times I said I'd make an appointment for her with an eye doctor, but she'd say no. Finally a few weeks ago, she agreed, so I made an appointment with Gary's Mother's doctor. She went along quite happily and the outcome was that it's not uncommon for cataract patients to form a film over the lens after surgery. He said it's an easily treatable thing. It calls for laser treatment and she'll be as good as new. We explained this to her and she said fine. The next day, I called to get her an appointment at the clinic and got one for today, the 17th. A couple days later, the clinic sent out an appointment card which I gave her. (BAD idea). I thought she'd keep it in her purse or somewhere and look at it every now and then to be reminded of when her appointment was. I also put it on the calendar. What I didn't consider is that when she gets anything with a phone number on it, she decides she has to call that number. She doesn't know why, but she insists on calling. So she started pestering Gary about calling the clinic. (The card said: "If you need to cancel, call...") He kept telling her that she didn't have to call, but it didn't do any good. He kept telling me I should never have given her the card – like I hadn't figured that out. He did finally talk her out of calling. This was on a Saturday. Sunday morning, she came in and woke us up at 6:00 a.m. to say that she had been trying and trying that number for over an hour and no one would answer. Gary took the card away and said I'd take care of it later. She asked me about it later in the morning and I tried to explain, but to no avail. After a while, she forgot about it, or at least stopped talking about it.

May 18, 1990

Guess what we found today?! $200! I took Mom out to the bank to take care of some stuff and on the way she said she had something special to tell me. Then she got all tangled up in her words, but I determined that she had found something that was packed away since she came from Roswell and she didn't want to tell me what it was. She wanted to show me when we got home, and didn't want anyone but me to know about it. After we got home, she said she had to find a place we could talk alone, away from Gary and David. We went into her room and she told me to go wait for her in the bathroom, which I didn't. She pulled this little make-up case out of the closet and led me back to the bathroom. She didn't want anyone (and at this she nodded over her shoulder to Dad's and the Pope's pictures) to hear. I insisted there was no one there except us, but she knew otherwise. In the bottom of this make-up case was an envelope with $220 in it. She had been concerned about it all day because she had no idea where it came from. She said she hadn't had that case out in YEARS but if anyone else knew about it they would undoubtedly claim it was theirs. You know Gary and David! I reminded her of the $200 she had lost about two months ago, but she didn't remember. I assured her it was hers, she could keep it, there was nothing shady about it, and no one else would try to claim it. She's been going around now for the past couple of hours being relieved over and over again each time it comes into her mind. I told her to put it back in the case if she wanted to and that I'd remind her it was there whenever she needed money.

But I'm digressing from yesterday's story. The interesting thing about tonite's little incident is that I was the only one she would trust. After what happened Wednesday, I'm surprised.

A week or two after the appointment card business, I came home from work and she was out the front door as I got out of the car – not a good sign. She had an envelope and was all flustered. It was a Blue Cross/Blue Shield statement of a bill they had paid and I told her that, but she said that wasn't the problem. With the statement was a blank claim form which they send with every mailing just so you have them on hand. She was all upset because she didn't know how to fill it out. I explained to her that she didn't have to fill it out. It was just something for her to keep. She didn't buy that, but she let it go for a bit. As the evening went on, she came back to it half a dozen times. "I don't know how to fill this out. I don't know what a contract number is. I'm going to get in trouble if I don't fill this out." I told her in as many ways as I could think of that she needn't worry. It didn't have to be filled out, but the next time she got a bill, I would help her fill it out. I couldn't get it away from her to put it out of sight. (Sometimes she gets REALLY anxious about possession and you have to either back off or wrestle her for whatever it is). I thought maybe by the time I went to bed she'd accepted what I'd said. The next night I came home from work and she met me at the door with, "Well, I figured it out all by myself. I filled it out and I'm going to mail it." And being the mature, thoughtful, patient person I am, I snapped. I got furious. I said, "YOU DON'T HAVE TO

FILL THIS OUT!" and I took it and tore it in half. "YOU DON'T HAVE TO FILL THIS OUT!" and I tore it in quarters. "YOU DON'T HAVE TO FILL THIS OUT!" and I threw it in the trash. Then I went on saying things like, "Do you think I talk to you just to hear the sound of my own voice?! When I tell you something, I mean it. When are you going to learn to listen to me?" I was suddenly right back in the 70's when David and Michelle were little. With every word out of my mouth I knew full well it was pointless, stupid and mean. But did that stop me? No, of course not. I went upstairs after a while to put some stuff away and after a bit, she followed and said, "I'm sorry," in a very little voice. I said I was sorry too for hollering at her, but that she had to learn to trust me. I told her that if I tell her not to worry, she really doesn't have to worry. And that was that. Or so I thought.

Last Friday night, I had gone up to bed and I heard Mom talking at some length to Michelle. Later, Michelle came up and said Mom went through this long song and dance about some insurance thing. Fortunately, David had filled her in on it previously or she wouldn't have had a clue what Mom was trying to tell her. Anyway, the bottom line was that she told Michelle she still didn't believe me and she was going to do something about it. I asked if she had pulled the pieces of paper out of the trash, but Michelle said no. However, she still had the envelope and she was going to write to them and straighten things out. So I told Michelle to go along with it and offer to mail the thing for her and then just get rid of it, which is what I should have done in the first place if I had half a brain in my head.

I didn't hear anything more about it and Michelle left for Michigan on Tuesday, so maybe it was forgotten. Wednesday night, just before I went to bed, I said to Mom that I would be home from work about 8:45 the next morning to take her to the doctor. She said, "To go where?!" I said the eye doctor. She said, "You've been telling me all along that you didn't want me to go there!" I said no I hadn't and that it was on the calendar all along. I reminded her what it was for and she begrudgingly said okay, she'd go. I went to bed then. About 15 minutes later, Gary got home and I heard her say to him, "Do you get the feeling something is going on around here?" She asked him twice and he asked what she was talking about. "Well, Patty is trying to get rid of me." I almost fell out of bed. He said I wasn't, but she said she knew all the signs. Gary just came upstairs at that. (His method of dealing with her is to walk away in hopes that she'll forget). Meanwhile, David was trying and trying to tell her that I really was just going to take her to the eye doctor and we'd come right home afterward. She wouldn't buy that at all. She kept saying things like, "That's what SHE says too. I know what's going on. But I guess I'll just have to go along with it for now." Gary went back downstairs and just a couple minutes later came back up to change his clothes. As he got to the top of the stairs, I guess Mom figured he was coming up to appeal to me on her behalf because she called up to him not to go to any great trouble on her account. She'd deal with it herself. I told him to go right back down and talk to her since she seemed willing to talk to him, but he wouldn't. David was still plugging away with no success. Finally she went to bed in a very resigned, depressed, dejected manner. David came up and said, "She's going to have her bags packed when you come home tomorrow, you know."

As I expected, she hardly slept all night. The next morning I thought I'd see her up before I left for work at 6:00, but I guess she didn't want to see me because she never came out of her room. When I came home later, she was all dressed and ready to go – willing, but quiet. ON the way, she talked a lot, about everything but the issue at hand. The total time we spent at the clinic was maybe an hour, and during that time, she asked everyone who came near her if she had to stay, and couldn't she go home. The nurse and receptionist and doctor and assistant kept telling her the treatment would only take a few minutes, but she kept asking. She had no problem with the laser treatment. That didn't phase her in the least. It took about 20 minutes and she said later it was easy. But boy, was she happy to get out of there! The treatment was such that her vision improved immediately. She kept raving about that. That evening at dinner, David said, "Now do you believe me that Mom was just taking you to the eye doctor?" She said of course she did. He said, "Well, why didn't you believe me last night?" She seemed to get a little flustered and just said, "Oh well…"

The whole thing was just so weird. All along people have told me – and I've told myself – that I should just tell her whatever it takes to keep things running smoothly. But I keep trying to tell her the truth about everything. I just keep thinking that if I tell her the truth all the time, good or bad, she'll know she can trust me. But guess what? It ain't necessarily so! Turns out that there are times we haven't the faintest idea of how she's seeing or interpreting things. Somehow, the appointment card, the claim form and the eye appointment all got tied together in her mind along with heaven knows what else and look what came of it. Truth is not a concept with her anymore if she can't understand. Even now I find myself thinking that she'll learn from this incident and it won't happen again. But it seems as if her life is a series of isolated little time periods that have no connection to one another.

May 18, 1990

Other things she's forgotten; how to wash her hair and, frequently, how to tell time. I take her to the hairdresser now every Monday to get her hair washed and set. By the end of a week, believe me, she needs it. Her hair always looks nice, but she goes nuts with hairspray. Now and then, she can automatically tell the time. More often than not she has to think about it at some length, and sometimes she'll say something like, "It's six at the top and five at the bottom." (That was at 7:00 one evening). As far as the mail is concerned, we're going to get a post office box. That way, we can filter the mail before it gets to her. As an added bonus, maybe all our mail will get to us in a timely manner. Our mailman loses mail on a regular basis.

When I talked to Virginia, I had her put Bill on the phone so I could get sympathy. I've had shingles for the past three weeks or so and Gary said Bill would feel sorry for me because he had them once. Well, fat lot of good that did! Bill said he's been told that he had shingles when he was around 7 years old. No empathy there. This started when my left eye was itching unmercifully one day. Naturally, I rubbed it a lot and the next day it was red. It felt like I had a bug bite in the corner of my eye. I went to the medical department at work and they just gave me Neosporin which did nothing. The next morning, my eye was swollen and I noticed some 'bites' on the left side of my forehead and across the top of my head. I was horrified at the prospect that some bug actually got on my face at night and marched across my head, lunching as he went. My eye was swollen the next two mornings also, but would go down as the day went on. I felt like I had banged the top of my head on something and like I had an ear infection on the left side. I thought it was weird that all these things happened at the same time. On Monday, I talked to a clinic doctor at work and he said it didn't look like a bug bite to him, but it could be. Then I said, "Sure it is. See, I have a whole string of them across my head." As soon as I made the motion across the left side of my head with my hand, he said, "That's shingles!" I went to my own doctor Monday afternoon. He was taking down all the information I gave him about the previous five days and when I showed him the line of 'bug bites' with my hand, he had the same instantaneous reaction the other guy had. He said, "That's not bug bites; that's shingles!" He said there wasn't anything they could do for it. I'd just have to put up with the pain for a few weeks. The itching would subside when the rash went away. His concern was about my eye. He sent me to an eye doctor right then and there. That doctor told me that my eye wasn't affected at the moment, but if the virus got into the optic nerve, it would have to be treated early. There is no way to prevent it from happening. Since then, the rash and itching are almost gone. The pain is like an intermittent stabbing sensation on the left side of my head, but it doesn't last too long at a time. Up until yesterday, the top of my head was very sensitive to touch. It hurt if a breeze blew my hair! Yesterday and today, the stabbing, burning sensation is less, but I have a dull aching pain around my eye and in my forehead. This is getting genuinely boring. The eye doctor gave me drops for when the itching was most severe, but the rest of it is just there.

May 21, 1990

The eye doctor says my eye looks perfectly fine. He says the pain around it is nothing to worry about. I don't have to go back for two months unless something weird happens in the meantime.

I also had to go see Aunt Mary's lawyer today to finalize the will, tie up loose ends and write checks. In the course of all this business, the court had to appoint a *guardian ad litem* to represent Aunt Anne and sign a waiver for her. It couldn't be Jerry or myself because we have an interest in the will. So it was just a random attorney the court appointed. Since Aunt Anne doesn't make any sense, they don't have to talk to her. This guy's job consisted of being told the circumstances of the will and Aunt Anne's condition, and then he signed the waiver. For that he got $300. Not too shabby for five minutes of his time!

May 22, 1990

Yesterday, Gary was going to make meatloaf for dinner. He took a couple pounds of ground beef out of the freezer and stuck it in the microwave for a few minutes to defrost. Then he pulled off the defrosted part, put the rest back in the microwave and came upstairs to do some work. When he went back down, the defrosted meat was gone. Mom said it looked like something that had gone bad so she threw it away.

Today Michelle called me at work to say that Mom wanted to call me to ask if she could open my mail. I had a letter from St. Mary's Hospital and she was sure it was about her. I told Michelle to tell her it was probably something about Aunt Mary. Michelle went out shortly after that and sure enough, Mom was right on the phone. (She knows my number at work and uses it often). When I got home, I opened the envelope and it turned out to be the minutes of my last Human Investigation Committee meeting.[1] She was all over me to find out what it was, so I told her and, lest she doubt, I showed it to her. She tried to read it, but couldn't make heads or tails out of it. She said it was disgusting, using all those big words that no one could understand. Gary assured her that I could understand them, but she wanted me to tear it up and throw it away because we shouldn't have something like that in the house. Oh well ...

---

[1] *I was a 'citizen' representative on a board at a local hospital which reviewed research study protocols.*

May 27, 1990

Life gets stranger ... We now have a post office box. I figured that would solve the problem. Up until now, she never bothered with our mail. I brought the mail home Friday and a couple of items got left on a living room table. Just a little while ago, she started going through the stuff on the table including a computer notebook that a friend had brought over for Gary. She asked Gary if he knew where there was some money. Then she made a couple of other comments which we didn't understand at all and kept looking through his computer book. He told her there was no money in there. She said, "Sure," and kept looking. She dozed off a while later and when she woke up, she said she was going to bed. She gathered up Gary's mail and headed for her room. I told her that was Gary's but she said she had to read it over. She had the booklet with the Shamrock Marathon results in it and I let her keep that because he had two, but I took a receipt and a letter from her. She tried to take them back, but I wouldn't let her. She said, "Those are mine." I told her they were Gary's; that one was a receipt for a car part. She insisted the other was a letter to her and she had to have it. It told her it was from a mower repair place and as I could recall, she hadn't had her lawn mower tuned up lately. She looked at me as if I were an idiot and finally went on to her room. I told Gary he couldn't leave anything around any more. Say! This could be a bonus for me. For those of you who have never been here, Gary has this – up until now – unbreakable habit of leaving all his junk on the bottom two or three stairs. We've all gotten used to going around it on our way up and down stairs; in fact, quite some time ago, I even gave up trying to get him to move it when we have company. I don't think the kids ever remember seeing the right-hand side of the lower steps in all their lives.

We nearly put the finishing touches on our bedroom today. It really looks great. We had a rather small closet over the stairway and Gary built us a large one on the opposite end of the room. Then he took the door and walls out in front of the old closet and built a huge desk in the alcove with bookshelves above it. We painted the room yellow with a bit of navy blue here and there for accent. We got a navy blue rug which looks nice, but I figured out REALLY quickly that it will show every little bit of lint. Now we just want to get a ceiling fan.

Mom hovered through every step of the remodeling. It was quite interesting today trying to put the rug down while trying to keep her from standing on it. When it was finally in place, I brought the vacuum cleaner up and vacuumed it in about five minutes. It was all she could do to control herself. A proper vacuuming can take up to two hours or more – especially if you can't stand the vacuum cleaner marks and spend all that time trying to get rid of them. If you can't vacuum in just such a way as to eliminate all the lines, then you take a hand vacuum or a brush or broom and get them out. And heaven help the first person to walk on the carpet after this undertaking. A couple days ago, she vacuumed the carpet downstairs and David was the unfortunate who walked across it first. She told him to walk backwards over his tracks to get rid of them.

Mom is beginning to think Michelle, as house guest, is kind of overstaying her welcome. Her room is a mess, she doesn't go to bed till all hours, and she eats! How unruly can one get? Mom asked her today when she was leaving and suggested she leave early so as not to be driving after dark. Wait till she finds out Michelle is here for three months.

May 28, 1990

Memorial Day – three years ago today, Dad died. Look what he missed. I suppose there is some logic here. There's no way he could have dealt with this. Last night David and Michelle were getting ready to go to bed about 3:00 a.m. when they heard Mom. Michelle went to see what she was doing. She came out all dressed, but with her hair up in bobby pins. Michelle told her to go back to bed, but she said 'he' woke her up. She asked Michelle to go into her room with her, so she did. The bed was all made up. Michelle turned it down and asked if she had a nightgown. Mom didn't know. Michelle finally figured out that Mom was nervous about a picture of the Pope that was over the head of her bed. It's a framed photo that was taken when the Pope was in Phoenix and Tim[2] sent it as a gift for Mom. Mom has loved it all along, but suddenly she was sure it was watching her and she wouldn't undress or go to bed while it was there. David took it down and put it in the living room. She finally said she'd go back to bed so Michelle left. This morning she was really out in space. She slept a lot in the chair and didn't seem able to connect with us when she was awake. I think part of the problem was the fact that we were all home. She has no idea what day it is.

A little while ago, David and Michelle went out to clean up some branches in the back yard. She went out to help them so I took the opportunity to check out her room. Everything was neat and tidy as usual and I found a little stash of Gary's mail. I took the important stuff and left the rest where it was. I guess we're going to have to be a little more careful from now on. We keep saying, "But she's never done that before." New surprises every day.

Later that same day ...

It's been a rough day. I thought things were getting better as the afternoon went on, but apparently not. Mom hasn't been able to figure out all day where she is. She asked Gary to take her home when he goes; she told Michelle she knew who I was and who David is, but not who she (Michelle) is; she asked me if we would be leaving for home soon because she didn't want to be on the road after dark. She asked if it was Monday and I said yes. She said, "That's okay then, but we have to get home by Sunday." We all tried to tell her we were home and we all live here. Gary even sent her into her own room thinking she'd know where she was if she saw it. A little while ago, she decided we were just staying here for a while. She's been trying to get me to borrow one of her nightgowns ever since. When I told her I was going to bed, she got upset because I wasn't going into her room. She followed me upstairs and told me this wasn't my room, it was that other guy's room. I said it was mine and the other guy's and she accepted that, but still insisted that I borrow a nightgown. I said no and she finally went back downstairs, but not before she found and took my sewing kit. I let her. This is definitely not an evening to make waves. Just now she came back and asked which nightgown I said I wanted and I sent her away again. Should be a challenging night.

Earlier today, she asked me if I was ready to end this farce. I said sure, what did she want. She wanted her comb. I told her to look in her purse and her bathroom and off she went. I went outside to clean some porch furniture and when I came back in about 20 minutes later, she had her purse and make-up case over her arm and was on her way out the front door. She did say goodbye before she went out, though. I followed her out and asked where she was going. She looked confused for a minute and said she was going to find a comb and set off down the sidewalk. I called her back in and told her to go look in her bathroom. While she did that, I looked in her purse and pulled out the comb. I took it in to give it to her and she was satisfied, but I got the distinct feeling that she was suspicious about where I might have gotten it.

[2]*Tim is one of Carole's sons.*

June 4, 1990

Well, everything is back to "normal" now. Last Tuesday, Mom was rather more in touch than she had been on Monday, and by Wednesday, she was back to her typical, confused self. David thinks the whole thing had to do with it being the third anniversary of Dad's death. He may be right. This is sort of the way she was when we got home from our trip to Maryland at Thanksgiving. For a day or two, she was totally lost. In that case, we assumed it was just too much confusion and stimulation. I kind of get the feeling that these have been little previews of what's ahead, because her behavior under the circumstances was very much like that of Aunt Anne. She's out of touch all the time now.

Gary left a postcard from the dentist sitting on a living room table a couple days ago. It was a notice for an appointment on June 22. Mom decided it had something to with Aunt June.[3] I tried to explain, but she couldn't figure out what Gary and our dentist had to do with her sister. I hid the card when she went into the kitchen for a minute and she forgot about it.

Aunt June, is your birthday this month? A couple days after she saw the postcard, she told me she thought it was your birthday and I wasn't sure if the card triggered that thought or if she really remembered. Every now and then she'll mention something she remembers and it turns out to be true, but I'm never sure when to believe her. A street sign or something will cause her to remember something specific from the past, and on the other hand, she'll quite seriously say something like, "This fellow went to Blessed Sacrament with me," and she'll be pointing out Richard Crenna in the TV book.

[3] *Aunt June is Mom's oldest sister. She lived in Georgia at the time these letters were written. (And her birthday is in June!)*

June 9, 1990

Aunt June, I got your letter the day I was mailing out the last installment, and believe me, I was delighted to get it. It's a real boost to get moral support from any source. Aunt Mary used to tell me the kind of things you wrote in your letter, and I really missed hearing it. Thanks.

I heard from Uncle Jim yesterday.[4] He called to see how Mom was doing which I couldn't get into in detail because she was sitting right there, so I put her on the phone so he could kind of judge for himself. He said he was going to come take her out for lunch next Wednesday. I was really pleased that he actually made a date to come over. I've contacted a few of her friends and they've all said they'd be in touch, but that's as far as it went. Aunt Nan's away for a while again so that just leaves me. Even Gary, David and Michelle never take her out. They're real patient about having her live here, but they still come and go as they did in the past. Except for going to work, I can't step out the door without her wanting to come along. If I take her with me, every trip becomes a major project. If I go without her, I feel guilty. If I stay home, either I'm annoyed because Gary, David and Michelle are free to go out, or I choose to stay home and she pesters me to go out. I try to put myself in her place – I know that I'm her only source of transportation and entertainment – but rather than making me more sympathetic, it just makes me aggravated.

Here's a bright note. I went to a Caregiver's Seminar this past Wednesday night and I had occasion to meet a woman around my age who lives nearby and whose mother has Alzheimer's. She moved in with her mother three years ago. From what I could tell, her mother is at about the same stage as Mom. I've been to three support group meetings and one other Caregiver's Seminar, but the majority of the people are older folks taking care of a spouse. It's interesting to hear someone else echo the same kind of things that are going on around here. The key difference, however, is that her mother knows and admits that she has Alzheimer's and on occasion, jokes about it. But she does a lot of the same things as Mom – roots around in the trash, hides things in her room, alternately thinks that she's broke or that people are stealing her money, gets all mixed up on the phone, and can't deal with mail. I thought it would be an advantage for this woman to still be in her own home where she has friends and neighbors nearby, but her daughter said that doesn't seem to matter. Her friends have all gradually dropped away because of her mother's strange behavior. The neighbors alternately don't want to deal with her or think the daughter is treating her badly because of the things the mother tells them – for instance, that she feeds her cold coffee and stale bread.

Remember that research project I told you about at UCLA? Well, I got a phone call from a research assistant a few days ago. I was quite surprised she called. She said the study is centered in the LA area because the participants would have to be there for at least a month. She said there have been a few people outside the area who were willing and able to spend a month there, but she said after the article was syndicated, they got something like 2000 inquiries from the LA area alone. The only other information she gave me on the study is that they have a grant for five years, so they will be tracking all the participants for at least that long.

Today hasn't been a terrific day. Earlier, I threw away an empty Kleenex box from the bathroom. A couple days ago, Mom bought a box of Kleenex and rather than put it in her own room, left it in the living room so everyone could use it. Unfortunately, Michelle doesn't realize that even though Mom says things like that, she doesn't mean it. What we buy is everyone's; what she buys is HERS! – unless, of course, she specifically offers it to you. For instance, she'll buy candy or ice cream and say it's for anyone, but unless she actually dishes up the ice cream and hands it to you, or hands you a piece of the candy, you had better not touch it. She hides candy in her room and would the ice cream too if it wouldn't melt. So

Michelle was observed using a Kleenex or two in the past couple of days. Yesterday, she left for Michigan for the weekend, so I guess she was fair game to be 'the accused.' Mom found the empty Kleenex box when she was going through the trash and got mad because Michelle had used HER Kleenex, even though she found that the one she put in the living room was still there. I got mad, mostly because she was rooting through the trash again, and also because she suspects David, Michelle or Gary whenever anything goes awry. She got upset and said I was mean to her and it went downhill from there.

[4]Uncle Jim is Mom's brother-in-law. His wife, Mom's sister Mary, died in 1988.

June 10, 1990

Another day, another approach . . . I had decided to go into work today to do a little catching up and, too, it's the one place Mom doesn't ask to go along. Actually, I did go to work, but I also went to the new mall afterwards and just wandered aimlessly and had an orange creamsicle yogurt with chocolate sprinkles. The miracle of chocolate! When I came home, I was ready to come home.

June 12, 1990

I took today off on a whim. I had to take Mom to the eye doctor this afternoon and I decided that rather than just take a couple of hours, I'd take the whole day and do whatever I felt like doing. I went out this morning at the regular time and as far as Mom was concerned, I was at work. My boss had said that if she called work, they'd just tell her I was not at my desk but that I'd be home in time to take her to the doctor. I bought myself a newspaper and went to a restaurant for a leisurely breakfast. Then I went to check out an adult day care center nearby. It really seemed nice. The woman I spoke to said they have about 15 to 20 people on any given day and about half of them are able to care for themselves and get around fine like Mom and half require very close supervision. It didn't seem like some programs that are set up more like nursery schools. I liked the place.

Anyway, from there I went to the library and sat around reading for a while. Then I went to the mall and didn't buy anything and eventually stopped for lunch. It was very relaxing.

When I got back, I took Mom to the eye doctor. He said the laser treatment worked just fine and she has nearly 20/20 vision in both eyes now.

June 22, 1990

Wednesday, Uncle Jim came to take Mom out to lunch. They called me at work because Mom was sure I'd rush right home to have lunch with them, and Uncle Jim said she had the idea that they were eating at our house. I told him he'd have a long wait because Mom doesn't cook, so he laughed and said they'd go out. They went to a restaurant on the lake and had a drink but the wait for a table got too long so they ended up going to another place. Uncle Jim marveled at the amount of food she can pack away. Then they went for a long drive and finally ended up at Aunt Nan's for a visit. That evening, I didn't come home from work because I had a hospice meeting at 6:00 and by the time I did get home around 9:00, Gary and the kids had gone out. I figured Mom would be all out of sorts being left alone and all, but she was in great spirits. She tried to tell me about her afternoon with 'that man' and wanted me to look up his phone number for her. I did that and she called him right up and asked if he'd come back the next day. He told her he had to paint his garage, but he'd see her again. I got on the phone then and he filled me in on their day and I assured him it did Mom a world of good.

Gary's been working night security at a golf club for the LPGA this past week. Yesterday he said he had a couple of rather strange messages on his answering machine at school. One guy from school called and said he wanted to know if Gary was all right. Then another woman called to see how sick he was and if he would be able to work on a project he's doing for her. He called the woman back and found out that she, and apparently others, had called our house, and Mom told them he was very sick and couldn't get out of bed. She had asked me early in the week what was wrong with Gary and I told her he was working nights and sleeping during the day, but apparently I didn't convince her. Most people know enough not to call here during the day unless they want to talk to her, but occasionally, someone new calls and I'm sure they hang up very confused as to what just took place.

Michelle had a boyfriend over for dinner tonite. This guy was coming from out of town and Michelle didn't know what time, so Gary, Mom and I went ahead and ate. Later, Gary cooked steaks for the kids. After they finished, they sat at the table for a while visiting. Then Michelle went to make a call to make plans to go to a movie with another couple. Her friend sat at the table waiting for her – that is, till Mom got up, went in the dining room and told him to get busy and pick up those dishes! He seemed a little embarrassed, but he did it and she went off to her room. David went and took the phone from Michelle and she went to help clear the dishes. I'll have to ask her later if she had forewarned this guy to expect just about anything.

CHAPTER 5

The need for supervision increases.

July 1, 1990

Carole, I got your card and books yesterday and I was so pleased! I loved the card! And the books are great. "The 36-Hour Day" is considered the 'bible' of Alzheimer's families and I hadn't had a chance to read it yet. Everyone has told me about it and I was going to go looking for it and now you've saved me the trip. The other one looks good too. I can't wait to get into them. But especially nice is knowing that you're thinking of me.

Last Saturday I asked Mom what she'd think about going to a senior citizen place once or twice a week. I told her it was a place where people went while their families were working. They get together to socialize and have lunch there and so on. She thought that sounded okay so I told her I'd take her over to see the place. When we arrived, there were six women there. It's pretty quiet on Saturdays and I figured it would be a good time for her to be there. The women were just finishing lunch. They came out, sat down and talked to Mom a bit while I was talking to the two women who were working there. It went rather smoothly, I thought; nothing startling or strange to scare her off. When we left, she said she didn't think she'd like to go there. I asked why not and she said she doesn't want to spend time with old people. She'd rather spend her time with young people. I told her those weren't the two options; that she would be going while we were at work, so it was either spend time with people her own age or spend more time alone in the house with no one to talk to all day. She said she couldn't go anyway because she had her things to do around the house (making beds, doing dishes, etc.) I told her the house was standing before she ever came and it would survive without her one or two days a week. She didn't seem convinced, and I didn't press the point. At least I've planted the seed. Whether or not she'll remember is something else again. I may insist she go one of these days, but we'll see. When the time comes that she can't be home alone, it will be easier to get her into the program full time if she's used to going part time.

Her speech patterns are getting tougher and tougher to understand lately. It used to be, even though she couldn't think of the right words, she'd say a word or phrase that would put you on the right track and you could kind of help her finish her thoughts. But more recently, there are times when none of us has the foggiest idea of what she's trying to say. Sometimes she'll go through this long speech at the end of which she says, "Okay?" and you don't know whether to say okay or not because you haven't any idea what you're agreeing to or what she might do. One day, I said okay and, as she gathered up her purse and headed out the door, I discovered I had just agreed to take her someplace.

Gary just got back from San Francisco Friday night. He had a real good time playing golf, running and going to baseball games. He is really grateful for the baseball tickets, Virginia. He said the seats were terrific. Susan, he found out about a restaurant in NYC that we have to try. One night he went to an excellent steak place. The manager of the restaurant asked him after dinner how he liked it and Gary said it was almost as good as Smith & Wolensky's in NYC. This fellow insisted it was better and said they have a restaurant in NYC also, and we'd have to try it next time we're there. He gave Gary his business card and wrote on the back, "Take good care of our friends." The name of it is Ruth's Chris Steak House.

July 2, 1990

Yesterday, Gary's mother came over and after dinner, Michelle's friend, Jill, came by. Shortly thereafter, Jill's boyfriend came over and we rented a movie, "New York Stories." During the first story, Gary's mother dozed off occasionally and Mom kept telling me we had better take her home, but Gary wanted to serve dessert first. He finally did that and afterwards he took his mother home. While he was out, David went out and

Jill's boyfriend left. When Gary got back, I went up to bed and he and the girls settled down to watch the rest of the movie. A few minutes later, Mom started asking where 'he' was. They told her he went home and David went out. She kept asking, but they weren't sure who she was talking about. Then she asked if they had his phone number because she wanted to call. Jill said she had her boyfriend's number, but that he was home sleeping. Mom insisted she call and get him on the phone because she wanted to talk to him. Gary told her no and she got all the more agitated. She started saying that she wanted to tell him to get home here right now. So they assumed she was talking about David. They said he'd be home soon. Then she started saying 'she.' Now they really didn't know who she was talking about. She kept asking where was she, what was her number, why wasn't she home, etc. So they thought maybe she was talking about Mrs. T. She was getting so upset that Gary finally told Michelle to call his mother and have her talk to Mom. She started talking like she thought Jill's boyfriend had taken Mrs. T. home and was up to no good (we were guessing). When Michelle got Mrs. T. on the phone, Mom said (almost hollering), "Is my daughter there!?" The conversation got fuzzier after that and Gary finally took the phone away and sent her upstairs thinking that maybe she was looking for me. When she came up here, she kept asking me about that other girl and how were we going to find her and get her home here. I tried to get her to see that all the people who lived here (and we named them one by one) were here, except David, and that everyone else was in their own home. She finally gave up and went downstairs. Michelle said she sat there for quite a while with her arms folded, looking angry. She asked one more time to get someone on the phone and then gave up. When David came in, she asked him a couple of off-the-wall questions and finally went to bed. Today, it's not even a memory, I guess.

July 7, 1990

NEWSFLASH!!! Mom's been married twice! She just told Michelle a little while ago. "My husband died, you know. He was very sick. We had only been married a couple of years." "No Grandma. You were married over 50 years." "We were? No, that was my first husband. I've been married twice." "What happened to the first one?" "Well, he was very sick too. And after the second one died, I decided that was enough for me. I wasn't getting married again." Three times is just too much, I guess. So there you have it – our two Dads.

Well, I've talked to Virginia twice since I wrote last and I've talked to Susan too. Fun! Virginia called the first time to make an offer to have Mom come out to Phoenix for a bit. But, quite frankly, I don't think she'd do too well. As you've gathered from things I've written, she doesn't respond well to change. First of all, she couldn't travel alone under any circumstances. Secondly, I doubt she'd tolerate the change in routine. Remember how she was after our trip to Jacqui's at Thanksgiving? She was absolutely in another world.

We're going to Philadelphia for a weekend the beginning of August and I've arranged to have her stay at Aunt Nan's. I'll be interested to see how it goes. The thing is, it's close by so Aunt Nan can bring her home if things get too hairy. I told Aunt Nan that I'd like to prepare Mom for the visit, but her reactions are so varied and erratic that it's hard to say what to expect. I also told her that Mom will probably ask where I am fairly frequently.

When Virginia called the second time, it was to say that she had just received a bucket full of melted chocolate and some soggy wrappers and she wanted to know what was originally in it so she could appreciate what she missed. Gary had sent her a bucket 'o' chocolate to thank her for the Oakland A's tickets. They assured him it would travel well even to a hot place like Phoenix, but guess what? Well, Gary's going to rattle their cage a bit and try to get restitution.

July 14, 1990

Dateline: 8 July 1990 – The Great Toilet Paper War! Mom goes into a panic Sunday morning and interrupts my shower to let me know she is out of toilet paper. All I had left was what was on the roll so I gave it to her. On the way home from Church, we stopped and bought six rolls. When we got home, I gave her two and put the other four in my bathroom. Later that day, she remembered she was out, but forgot that we bought more and asked me to take her to the store. I reminded her that we bought some, but she insisted we didn't. I told her to look in her room and she proceeded to search the whole house except for her room. She went through our dressers, Gary's camera bag, the stove, her purse, etc. etc. She'd stop every little while in frustration and beg me to take her to the store and I'd say no. Finally she did look in her room and didn't find the two rolls. She asked again if I'd take her to the store and I said even if I wanted to I couldn't because the only car here was David's and I can't drive that. She went searching again and this time found the four rolls I had taken upstairs. She marched downstairs full of accusations that I had taken her toilet paper and hid it on her. Fool that I am, I tried to explain it to her once more, but she was furious. Finally, I blew a gasket and told her to take every roll she could find in the house and quit bugging me about the blasted toilet paper. She threw the rolls she had in her arms down on the couch and started searching again. This time, she looked in David's car, in the refrigerator, under all the furniture, etc. After some time, she reappeared with two more rolls which she admitted to finding in the cupboard with the cereal. "And YOU put them there, didn't you?" I said. "Yes." "Now go put them in your room before you lose them again." "Okay." She did not, however, return my rolls to the linen closet. She would only concede to putting them on the stairs.

Tuesday night Aunt Nan called. Mom got to the phone before I did, but I picked it up upstairs a second later and listened to hear who it was. She was calling to invite Mom to lunch the next day, but the conversation started out with, "Guess who this is?" Mom didn't know and Aunt Nan kept trying to give her hints which confused her more. Finally Aunt Nan asked about lunch, but the question included the topics of lunch, shopping at the mall, the weather, and the time. By this time, Mom had no idea what she was talking about. (She was still back at the part about somebody being her brother Kernan's wife and why were they talking about someone who was dead?) I went downstairs then and Mom gave me the phone. Aunt Nan said she wanted to come over the next day, but Mom seemed reluctant. I told her to just come and that Mom would go with her gladly. Meanwhile in the background, Mom was saying "You make a date! You make a date!" When I hung up, I said Aunt Nan would be over to take her to lunch. She said,

"Now!?" I said no, the next day. Mom was still up when I went to bed. At about 1:30 a.m., I heard Michelle asking her what she was doing up. She told her to go back to bed. At about 3:30, I heard her up fixing breakfast. When I got up for work at 5:30, she was ironing. Then she called me at work at about 9:00 and asked why I hadn't come home to take her to lunch. I told her Aunt Nan would be over around 11:30. Shortly thereafter, Gary called to say Aunt Nan had to cancel. When he told Mom, she seemed relieved that she didn't have to sort out this lunch thing any more.

I remember an incident with Aunt Therese once. I was going over to their house to take her to a concert. When I got there, Aunt Anne was tearing her hair out. She had been trying and trying to get Aunt Therese to go up to the bathroom. What she was saying was, "Patty's coming over to take you down to the lake for an Irish concert, and it's going to last quite a while so you had better go to the bathroom before she gets here so you'll be ready and she won't have to wait." Well, Aunt Therese was lost after the first phrase and they were both at the peak of frustration when I came in. I said, "Aunt Therese!" and she looked at me. "Do you want to go out?" She smiled and nodded. "Then go to the bathroom." She went right up. Now I'm rediscovering with Mom – too many words and everything becomes a blur.

July 15, 1990

We took Mom to an RPO concert in Geneseo Friday night. They were playing the 1812 Overture including cannons and fireworks. Before they got to that, they played several other classical pieces. At the intermission, Mom wanted to go home, but I told her they hadn't played the 1812 yet and that's what we'd come to hear. She sat patiently for about ten minutes and then said, "I think I'll go home anyway." I didn't answer her right away. She looked around and noticed Gary was gone and said, "Well, I guess I won't, huh?" I thought she'd ask again after that, but she didn't. After the intermission, they played one other piece of music and then got into the 1812, so it wasn't too long a wait, fortunately. When they got near the end, I pointed out the cannons to her so they wouldn't take her by surprise. The ending was spectacular as always and she loved it. I asked her later if she was glad we stayed and she said she certainly was. The only minor mishap was that the instant they stopped playing, she was up, with her chair folded, told me we had to get going and as I turned to get my chair, she darted off into the crowd – in the dark. I took off after her and found her in rather short order, just in time to see her at the edge of panic. Disaster circumvented.

Remember I told you some time back how she would hassle the kids whenever they had their friends over for more than about half an hour at a time? Well, she hadn't done that in quite a while – until Friday night. When we got home from the concert, Michelle and two of her friends were watching a movie. We said hello and went on to bed. I thought Mom did too. Shortly afterwards, David came in with two of his friends and they were all watching TV. About 1:30 in the morning, I thought I heard Mom's voice. Gary woke me up and said, "Your mother's pestering the kids again," whereupon he went downstairs. She was trying to get them all to leave, even David and Michelle. Gary said she was shaking her watch at them and at one point actually took Jill by the arm and tried to get her up off the couch. It took Gary a good ten minutes to get her into her room – she argued all the way. Then he stayed downstairs for a while to be sure she didn't come out again – but of course, she did. When she realized he was still up, she slipped into the kitchen and puttered around and finally went back to bed. David took the whole thing in stride; he usually does. He's terrific about these things. Michelle wasn't so philosophical. She's more like Gary. She knows full well that Mom has a problem, but part of her still expects semi-normal behavior.

August 6, 1990

It's been quite a while since I had a chance to sit down and write some more. We just got back from our weekend in Philadelphia last night. Mom stayed with Aunt Nan. But I should backtrack and fill you in on the past couple weeks.

Well, I just took a 7 hour break. At the end of the last sentence, Mom came up and asked me for ice because she banged her head on a cupboard door. I went down and got some ice out of the freezer and put it in a plastic bag. After a few minutes, when it started to melt, she got all flustered over that and spent the next half hour or so going back and forth between her bathroom, the kitchen and the living room trying to solve the dilemma. I think at this point she had forgotten about her head. Each time she'd come by me, I'd tell her to dump the bag and get another ice cube and wrap it in a washcloth. She'd say okay, but she never did it. Finally, about half an hour later, she came out with a big patch of kleenex taped to her head with bandaids and a white linen handkerchief that she held to her head. I must have looked surprised because she said, "Oh, it doesn't hurt any more, but it's still wet." About half an hour after that, she dismantled the whole thing. What a project!

About our weekend away, I had asked Aunt Nan some time back if she'd be willing to take Mom and she readily agreed. We decided we wouldn't tell Mom till the last minute. On Wednesday, I finally got up the nerve to break it to her. My stomach had been in knots leading up to this because I just knew she'd object. So I brought up the fact that Gary and the kids and I were all going to be away for the weekend and how would she like to spend the weekend with Aunt Nan. Well, much to my surprise, she said, "I think I'd like that." She said she didn't want to be alone and thought it was a good idea. Phew! But then she spent the next hour or so asking me what day it was and what day we were going away and how many days away was that and what day it was and what day we were going away and how many days away was that and what day it was . . . you get the idea. Thursday I came home from work early to get things ready. I was doing some ironing and she was watching (from about 2 inches away). I asked her if she had her stuff together to take to Aunt Nan's. She said no, so I suggested she do that and she'd need enough clothes for three days. She asked for what and I reminded her of the weekend with Aunt Nan. She said, "I'm not going anywhere!" I told her she was and recounted our conversation of the night before. She said, "I'm not going over there! I'm not leaving this house!" So I said (firmly, trying not to lose my temper), "Let me put it this way. You don't have a choice. We are going away and you're not staying here alone." She still said no, but with a little less emphasis. So I repeated, "You don't have a choice. I'd suggest you get your things together or I'll have to do it for you." Gary came in shortly later and I told him to go in her room and offer to get down her suitcase, which he did. She was all bright and cheerful with him. A while later (she had been in her room for some time), I called her out for dinner. She came out and said to me, "I'll tell you what. Why don't you and I stay home this weekend?" I said no and she dropped it. Friday morning, I intended to take her over at 9:00. As soon as I got up, I could tell she was more in space than usual. I was having a hard time communicating with her. About 8:00 I asked if her things were ready. She gave me a vague answer and went into her room. I followed her in and, lo and behold, she had actually packed! She was distant for the next hour, but agreeable. Just before we were to leave, she got a box and started gathering all sorts of junk to take along – pins, paperclips, toothpicks, etc.

August 10, 1990

I let her gather all her treasures and put them in the suitcase and off we went. When we got to Aunt Nan's, I took her suitcase upstairs. She came along willingly and Aunt Nan chatted away trying to make Mom comfortable. When we went back downstairs, I stood and talked with Aunt Nan a few minutes and then said, "Well, I'd better go. I'll see you after the weekend." Mom looked as though I hadn't said a word. So I left. She didn't follow or say anything, but when Aunt Nan followed me out to the car, she suddenly appeared at the door. Aunt Nan went back and gave her a hug and maneuvered her back into the house.

I came back to pick her up Monday morning and her first comment was, "Oh! Oh! Oh! You've forgotten all about your family!" Aunt Nan said the weekend went pretty well till Sunday. All that day, Mom kept asking to go home and it was a bit of a task to put her off. In fact, Aunt Nan finally called our house about 7:00 p.m. just so she could tell Mom we weren't home and guess what? We were. We had gotten back earlier than expected so I told her to tell Mom she got the answering machine. She said okay, she'd see me in the morning and hung up.[1] Afterward I thought that was kind of a dumb thing to say because Mom doesn't know what an answering machine is, let alone that we have one now.

We just bought the machine a few days ago because Mom gets so upset when she gets calls during the day. She calls me at work looking for Gary and wants to call all over looking for him. So now we turn on the machine and turn off the phones when we're out. Now that we've solved the mail problem and the phone problem, anyone got any ideas on how to solve the trash problem? She's getting worse about going through the trash. The other day when I got home from work, she took me aside 'secretly,' pulled my bedroom waste basket out from behind the couch, took me out on the back porch and showed me all the stuff that was in it – some ads, empty envelopes and, horror of horrors, six baseball hats. (Gary has tons of them and threw a few away). She wanted me to go through the papers and keep them and to give the hats to 'the kids.' I asked what kids, but she ignored the remark and tried to get David to give them to 'the kids.' I told her the hats were dirty and we couldn't give them away, but she didn't buy that either. She went off with them and I haven't seen them since. Oh well. A couple days later, Gary came home and found her in her room with the contents of our waste basket all over her bed. I suppose it's a plus that she doesn't throw things away randomly, but this is ridiculous. In fact, if I have anything I don't want her to see, I have to take it to work to throw it away.

[1] Aunt Nan was really sweet about it, but made it clear after their weekend together that she never wanted to do that again. It's a whole different ballgame after having watched Alzheimer's 'from the outside,' to get up close and personal. It's something you just can't explain to people unless they've been through the 24/7 experience.

August 11, 1990

Gary and David went to Toronto for a Blue Jays game today and Michelle went to a concert with Jill. So I took some sausages out of the freezer for Mom and me and intended to make waffles since we had Bisquick in the cupboard. Come suppertime, I went to get the Bisquick out, opened it up and discovered there was no Bisquick in the box, just garbage. Apparently the last time Gary finished up a box, Mom managed to fish it out of the trash, fill it with other garbage and put it back in the cupboard. So much for waffles!

We had a real nice weekend in Philadelphia, by the way. Gary spent his weekend on baseball and golf; David on baseball, golf and baseball; Michelle visited one of her boyfriends and shopped; and I ate and shopped and ate and rested and ate and visited and ate and rested. It wasn't a wasted weekend.

August 15, 1990

All's quiet on the home front the past few days. Mom and Gary had a fight about whether or not she could make our bed on Sunday, but Gary won. He had stuff – including himself – all over the bed, because he was working on a student workbook he's writing. Mom stewed and grumbled and fretted all afternoon, but fortunately, Gary doesn't boil over as easily as I do, so it all worked itself out.

Yesterday when I got home from work, Mom showed me a bit of a tear in her bedspread and told me how she intended to fix it. I left her alone with it and she happily worked away at it for over an hour; plenty of time for me to fix dinner without her being about 3 centimeters from my elbow the whole while. It was great. The whole evening was virtually normal. Maybe I'll find her other things to mend.

Gary took the mothers to Church for the holy day today at noon so I didn't have to do that when I got home. All in all, a peaceful week.

CHAPTER 6

One year later and life takes on a semblance of routine.

August 19, 1990

I baked two rhubarb pies today. It felt like fall. Yesterday everyone was sweltering in the heat and today we're bundled up in long sleeves and sweaters with the house closed up. We had friends over for supper last night and I had made all cold foods because it was too hot to cook or to eat anything heavy. Today, we used the oven all day. That's what makes Rochester interesting, I guess.

Michelle is going back to school on Saturday. School doesn't start till the day after Labor Day, but she has band camp for a week before that. Tuesday, David is going to Toronto for a couple of weeks for work. Any time he's traveled for work before, it's been to little 'nobody every heard of them' towns. Gary is going to go up for a ballgame while David's there.

We had Mrs. T. over for dinner today. Mom and Gary got into an argument over making the bed again. Same as last week – he had all his papers all over. Only this time, he came downstairs for a break and she scooted upstairs. He called up to David to head her off at the pass, but David is no match for Mom when she has a mission. So Gary flew up the stairs just in time to find her shuffling all his papers into a heap.

August 23, 1990

Last night Gary fixed us hot dogs for supper about 6:30 p.m., but he didn't eat just then because he wasn't hungry. Later in the evening, Michelle went out and got Mom some ice cream which she ate around 10:00. About 11:00 Gary fixed himself two hot dogs and sat down in the living room to eat them. He said Mom came over with her purse in hand and watched him eat – well, more like watched his plate – moving closer and closer till she was just about hanging over it. He said, "Would you like a hot. . ." and before he finished the question, she snatched his second hot dog off the plate and wolfed it down before he finished the first one. Then she went to bed happy. He said it was all he could do to keep from laughing out loud.

August 24, 1990

I came across another research study being done on the genetic aspects of Alzheimer's. This one was out of Duke University. I called to get more information, but in this case, even though it's a nation-wide study, you have to have two living relatives with Alzheimer's; that is, two who are related to each other. I think they're going to be hard pressed to find many people in that category.

September 1, 1990

Gary and a friend have gone to Boston this weekend to take all Michelle's stuff to her. They also planned to take her out to the Hard Rock Café for her birthday. My 'baby' is actually 21 today!

Last night I was watching TV and Mom was dozing on and off in her chair as usual. About 10:30 p.m. she woke up, got up and mumbled something and headed toward her room. I assumed she was going to bed, but she took a left turn and went into the kitchen instead. Then she came back through the living room and headed for the front door. I thought she was going to close it, but she went outside. I waited to see what she was going to do, but she didn't come right back, so I went to the door and turned the front light on. She was trying to get our car doors open, one after the other, but they were locked. I told her to come back in, but she didn't seem to hear me. So I went back and sat down. A minute or so later, I heard her footsteps fading away down the driveway. I went out and called to her but she just kept on going down the sidewalk. I went after her, caught up with her about three houses away and asked where she was going. She said, "I'm going to Church." I said, "No, you're not. You're coming home and going to bed." She turned right around then and followed me home. Once we got back, I had to tell her a couple of times to go to bed before it seemed to sink in.

Today, she's back to 'normal.' We went grocery shopping this afternoon. She's got a new fun thing that she does now. She examines other people's carts to see if they're buying anything interesting. If she sees something she'd like, she attempts to strike up a conversation to find out where they got it. Sometimes they understand her, sometimes they don't. Sometimes I try to get her to move along and leave people alone, and sometimes I don't.

It's been a year now since she's been here. It really doesn't seem that long – well, some days it seems like forever – but it's kind of surprising to think it's been a whole year.

September 4, 1990

Gary started back to school today – finally! He whined about it, but I made him go anyway. David started a new job today. He's done all his previous co-op sections at one company, Retrotech. He's only got this one fall section left so he thought he'd try something different. He's working for Fairport Electric. He'll go back to school in December and graduate in May. Doesn't seem possible.

After Mom's wandering off in search of Church in the dark Friday night, it's been a rather uneventful weekend. Gary came home from Boston late Saturday night. They had a real good time, but he said (as was reported on a Boston traffic report) it looked like there had been a major furniture explosion all over the city. College kids were moving in everywhere. Vans, trucks and U-hauls filled the roads. He said it was quite something to see. Saturday afternoon, they took Michelle out to the Hard Rock. Michelle made the mistake of telling the waitress it was her 21st birthday and shortly thereafter, the waitress came up behind her and tied two helium balloons in her hair. Her hair stood up in the air in two bunches. Then the music was turned off in the restaurant and a major announcement was made. Everyone cheered and carried on. She was properly embarrassed, but she left the balloons for a while. They were sitting right near the entrance and whenever folks waiting would stop and stare, she'd say, "What's the matter! Haven't you ever seen balloons before!?"

September 15, 1990

Well, it's been quite a while since I sat down here to write. Gary went to New Jersey last weekend for a golf tournament. A friend who lives in Pennsauken holds a charity golf tournament every September and Gary has gone down the last two years. He came back this year having won a 10-speed bike – not by his expert playing, mind you, but in a drawing. He said everyone decided the drawing was fixed though, because he had sold raffle tickets earlier in the day.

David's birthday was yesterday and I bought him a watch. Conveniently, he recently broke his other one and mentioned that where he's working now, there's no clock. Do you suppose these were subtle hints? I took Mom with me on a couple of shopping trips looking for the watch, but I was a bit concerned that she'd tell David that's what we were doing. At each store, I'd tell the sales clerk that I was looking for a gold men's watch for my son for his birthday. I needn't have worried though. I bought one last night and today she asked me why I wasn't wearing my new bracelet.

Mike & Debbie are coming over for supper in a little while so I'd better get going. It's always interesting to see what Mom will do when people are over. Last weekend, we had friends over on Sat. night and in the middle of the conversation, she asked me if she should bring up "the stuff" from the basement. I said no, even though I had no idea what she was talking about. But, true to form, she ignored me, went off and came back with a box of some of her older and more formal clothes that she doesn't wear any more. She proceeded to show them to our company. There was no talking her out of it and they were polite about it. Another time, when Jim & Sandy were here, she took off for her bedroom and came back with a pair of slacks that she insisted Sandy should have (as if anyone could wear her size fours!). I tried to stop her, but Sandy just said okay, she'd put them aside and take them home later. Then when they left, she conveniently 'forgot' to take them along.

Mike & Deb just left and the evening was uneventful for the most part. Initially, Mom kept going in her room and changing her shirt. She went from her Lake Tahoe sweatshirt to a blouse to a sweater (and came out carrying a sweatshirt), to her Manion Sisters sweatshirt before she settled down. I guess she just wanted everyone to see an array of her clothes.

Just before Mike & Deb left, I had gone upstairs. Mike asked for an auto coffee cup so he could take his coffee with him. I hadn't heard the request, but then Mom came upstairs. I heard her ask David if I was in the bathroom and then ask him something else he didn't understand. Next thing I knew, she was knocking on the bathroom door and trying to open it. I told her to leave the door shut. When I came out (hurriedly), she said, "They need cups, two cups!" At which point, I heard Gary call up for her to come downstairs; that they were all set. I started down and she got annoyed and pushed past me into the bathroom. When I got downstairs, they were on their way out the door and had the coffee in an auto cup. Mom then appeared with two paper bathroom cups and insisted on giving one to Mike and one to Gary. Like a genius, I was trying to explain to her that they had what they needed, and of course, she was ignoring me altogether. Mike, who had more wits about him than I did, just accepted the paper cup and went on his way.

Considering what I know and read and say, there's still this huge chunk of my brain that believes if I can just explain something to her, she'll understand; or if I can get her to use the right words, she'll remember them the next time. For instance, the other night, I had come up to go to bed. Gary was away and David was out. She came up to ask me if she should turn off the living room light. She couldn't think of the word 'light,' but after a few words and gestures, I figured out that that's what she was getting at. Rather than just tell her to leave the light on, I actually waited to see if she could come up with the right word and then when I said the word 'light' for her, I had her repeat it. The dumbest thing is, if I heard someone else go through this exercise with her, I'd know full well that it was a waste of time. Oh well.

By the way, Aunt June, I got your letter the other day and thank you. It's always great to hear from you. Do let me know when you move.

October 4, 1990

For those of you who don't know, I just spent five days in Phoenix thanks to Gary, Virginia's "Trips-R-Us" Travel Agency (motto – "If you got there on time, you didn't book it with us."), Bill's Limo Service (English speaking driver, baggage service), and Carole's Hotel/Spa/Country Club/Resort/Bed & Breakfast/Time-Share/Condo (busses welcome). What a great time! Ruth's Chris Steakhouse was superb!!

November 18, 1990

A new chapter – tomorrow I have to call a locksmith and get new locks on our doors that we can lock from the inside and the outside with a key. Last night, Mom was up at 2:00, 3:00, 3:30 and 5:30 a.m.. Twice she headed out the door. She was trying to get to Church. It had been suggested to me that we put a chain lock on the door, up near the top or down near the bottom. As long as it's out of immediate sight range, she wouldn't have the logic to look for it and open it. But that wouldn't help on nights when David and Michelle are out late.

November 23, 1990

We had a relatively quiet, but nice Thanksgiving. Michelle was home, but we didn't have anyone else here for dinner. Mrs. T. went to Sue & Ed's and Jerry & Marcy couldn't make it. After dinner, we went out to a movie and then David and Michelle went out with their friends. This morning, they both took off for Boston. David will be back on Sunday and Michelle will be home in about three weeks. Susan & Charlie didn't get to come up for the weekend. (Boo! Hiss!) We missed them.

I've been thinking and rethinking that lock thing. I'm not convinced that a double key lock is the answer. That would mean that during the day, we'd have to leave the house unlocked all the time while we're out or else Mom would be locked in. Not a great pair of options. Maybe I'll go back to the chain lock idea.

November 25, 1990

I've re-inherited dishwashing privileges. Lately, the arguments about Mom's not using soap to wash the dishes have been getting more and more frequent. I keep telling her that rinsing dishes and wiping them with a towel that just keeps getting grungier by the minute just isn't acceptable – that we're all headed for some wonderful kind of germs down the road. Her objective, it seems, is just to get everything out of sight, to keep the kitchen looking neat. It doesn't matter that dirty or greasy dishes are being put in the cupboards. She just doesn't want to see them on the counter. Another daily battle.

November 29, 1990

I just got back from another Caregiver's Seminar. This one was on Alzheimer's research. We thought it would be on medical research, but it was actually on research studies being done with caregivers and families. It was interesting, but it always seems to me that with these types of studies, all they do is run around in circles. They do these lengthy studies over months or years and when they get to the end, they say they 'think' they've found something out, but maybe not. Not much comes from the results anyway. For instance, one speaker tonight listed all these studies about stress, depression, anger, and family dynamics with regard to Alzheimer's. As it turns out, the majority of us in the audience could have told him the same things he found out without all the trouble of a study. One study concluded that women have more difficulty handling aggressive patients than men do; another showed that people with social supports do better overall than those without; and another showed that excess burdens cause stress. Makes you wonder how much time and money went into discovering the obvious, doesn't it?

Mom's getting fuzzier lately in the late evening and early morning hours. I've told you about the occasions when she would wander off if she had been dozing. Well, it seems like that half-wakeful state is occurring more often. She's still alert during the day (enough to argue with Gary when he tries to get her to stay out of the trash).

This past week, being Thanksgiving, there was someone home every day from Wednesday through Sunday. Mom expected it to continue, I guess, because the following Tuesday, when I came home from work, Mom was fit to be tied. "There wasn't a soul in the house all day; no one even came to the door." She apparently even went next door to ask the neighbors where we were and why she had been left all alone. Any change in normal patterns. . .

December 1, 1990

Now we need to find some skeleton keys to fit our upstairs rooms. The bathroom and bedrooms up here all have locks but no keys. Mom goes through our drawers now and then which I haven't done anything about because there's nothing in there to harm, but recently, she has taken a couple of things from David's room and we're concerned about his school work and all. She's not taking them to take them, but she MOVES things and it can be a real challenge to find them again. Every day, she empties the wastebasket and cleans up a little in the bathroom. Well, today, I discovered HOW she was 'cleaning up.' Apparently, she takes whatever is in the wastebasket and wipes the sink out with it. I won't tell you what I caught her wiping the sink with today, but I cleaned and disinfected the sink twice afterward.

December 8, 1990

Mom is trying to figure out this whole Christmas concept. She asked me to get her money from the bank which I did, but she's still convinced she doesn't have more than a few pennies. She's been rifling through her room finding things to give as Christmas gifts. She pulled out the kangaroo we brought her from Australia a couple years ago and she said she would give it to "the children." I asked her what children, but she had no idea. I've taken her shopping a couple of times recently, but she finds the prices of everything outrageous and won't spend any money. Then a couple days ago, she brought the kangaroo, a mechanical penguin, and a little stuffed dog to show me and said she had to have paper to wrap them because she was going to give them to me and Gary and David. (I guess I had better remind her about Michelle again). I think I'll take her shopping again tomorrow and see what happens. Maybe we'll go to Woolworth's.

December 14, 1990

Well, that didn't help much. Mom had read through all the ads in the Sunday paper and came across one for a drug store that had wrapping paper, 150 sq.ft. for $4.98 and she wanted to get some. We went out to the mall and went into Sears. She found wrapping paper there, 150 sq. ft. for $3.98 and insisted it was WAY too expensive. So she picked out a roll that was 50 sq.ft. for $1.99. (No, I didn't try to explain it to her – I let her buy it). But as we approached the counter, she found a $5 bill in her wallet and told the clerk, "Whoa, wait a minute! I can't pay for that!" I told her to give him the five and she just pointed to the price with an annoyed look. I told her $1.99 was less than $5.00. She was skeptical, but she gave the guy her money. He rang it up and gave her change. She spent a few minutes putting the change in her wallet and stood there waiting. Then she asked the clerk, "Now what?" He said, "You're all set. You can go now." She asked if he was coming too. He looked quite confused by this time, so I snatched the wrapping paper and herded her on down the aisle.

On the way home, she said she wanted to go to the bank again and get all her money out. I told her she couldn't and that she had plenty of cash for the time being. She insisted that she didn't, but I had been keeping track and knew she had about $170 to $180 squirreled away somewhere. Then came the accusations again of someone stealing her money. I told her when we got home, she was to look for her money till she found it. It took her about five or ten minutes to find it – $190 in three different places.

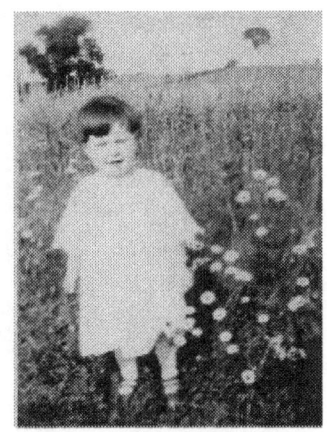

1914

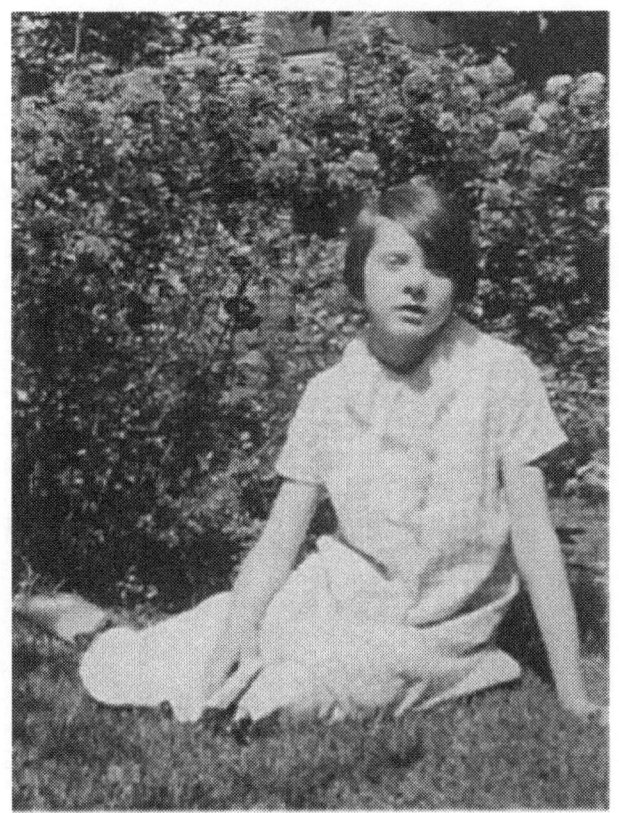

1924

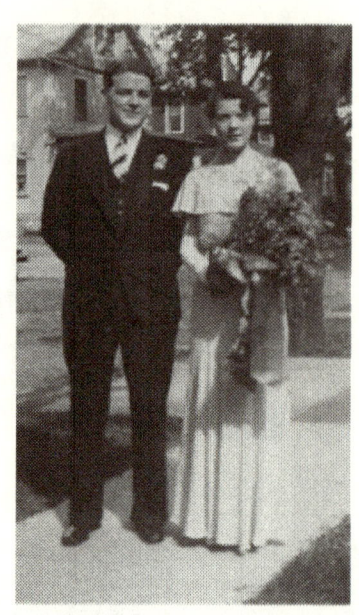

George & Bea 1932

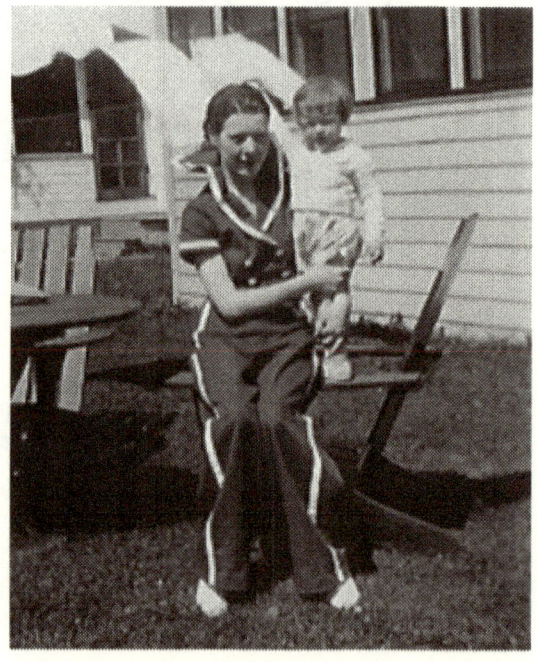

Bea & Carole 1935

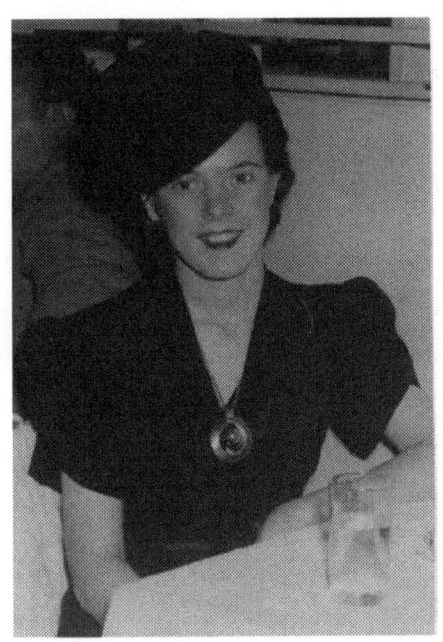

1935

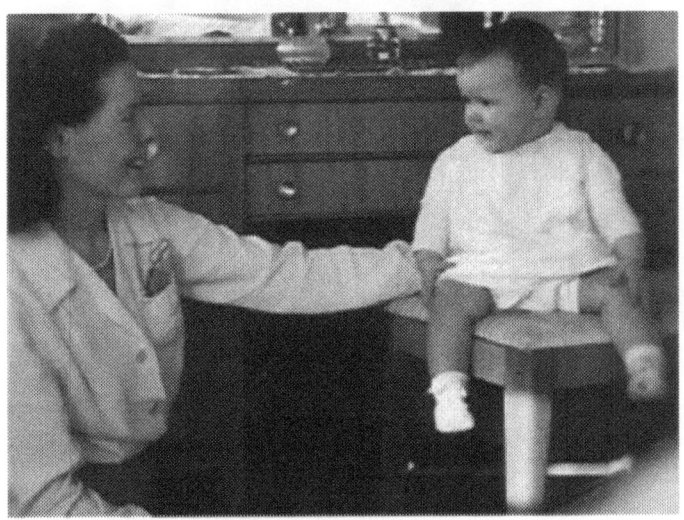

Bea & Susan 1944

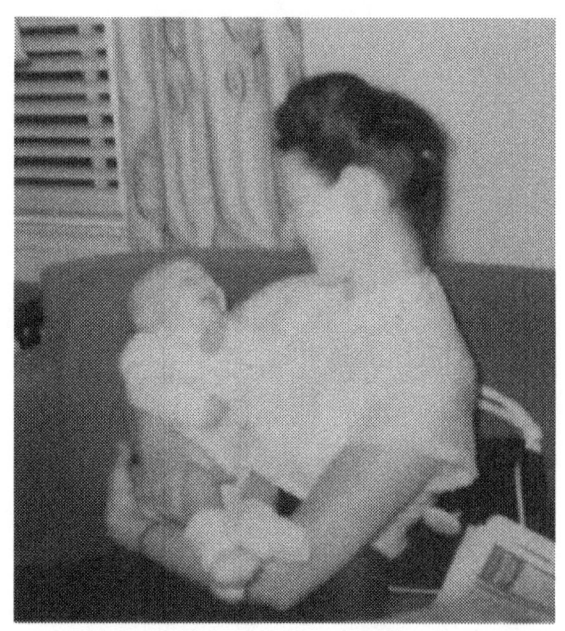

Bea & first grandson, Terry 1955

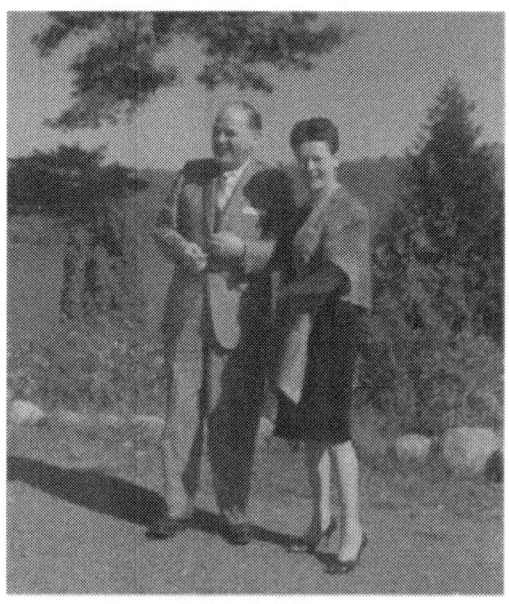

George & Bea, Adirondack vacation ~1960

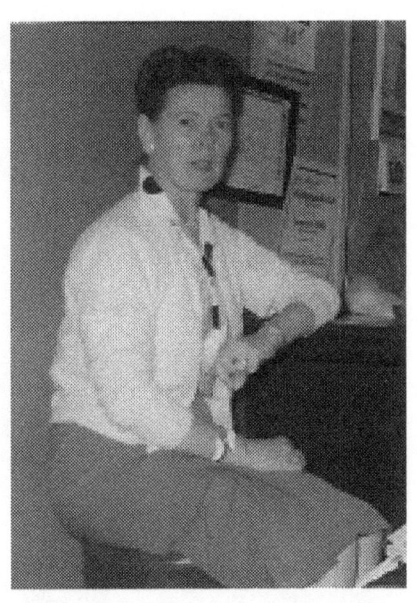

This was Mom's idea of 'dressing down' 1961

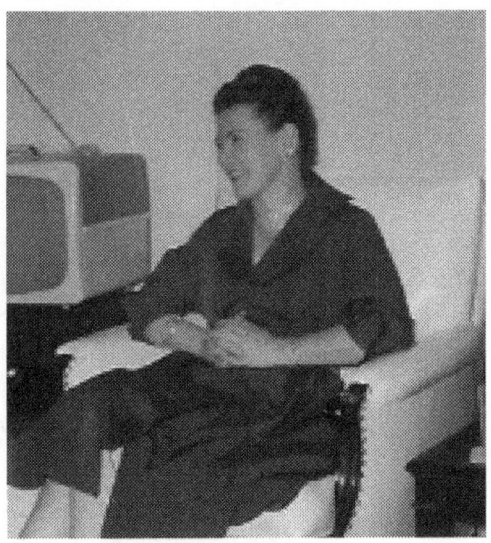

Relaxing at home; 1962

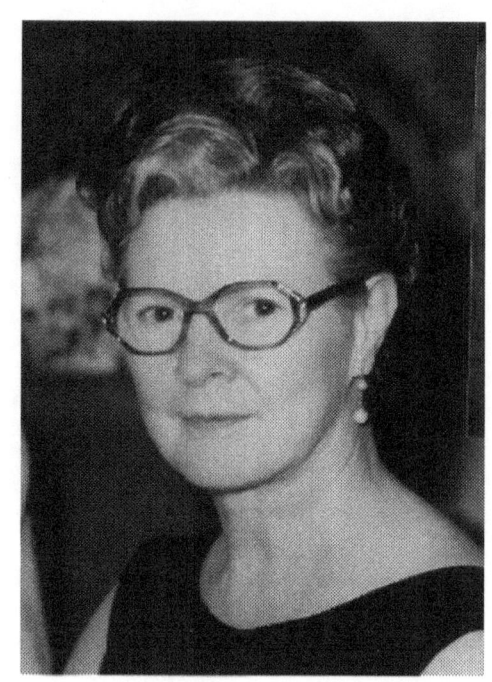

1978

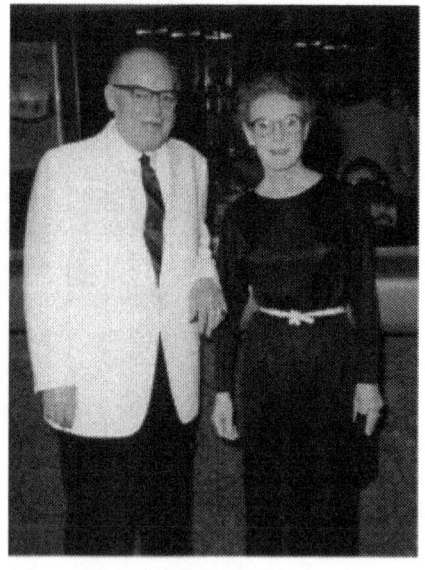

George & Bea on a cruise ~1980

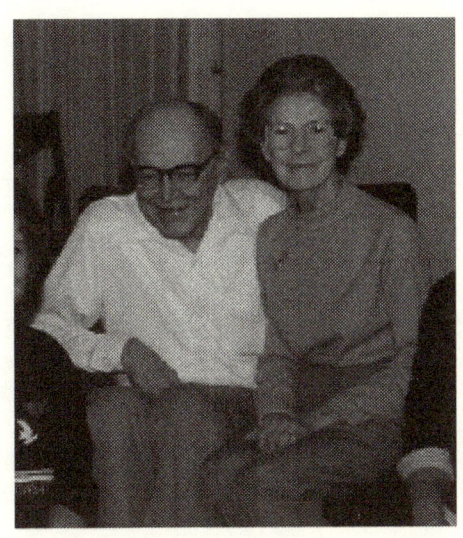

George & Bea, Roswell, NM, November 1986

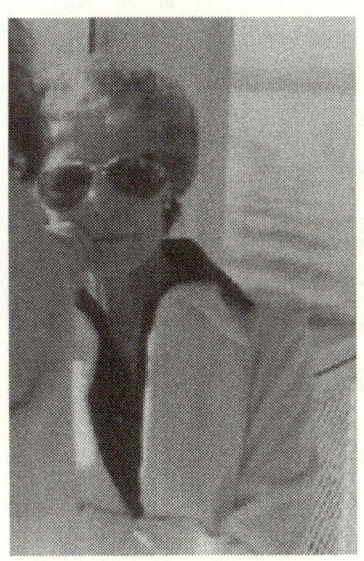

Lake Tahoe, August 1987

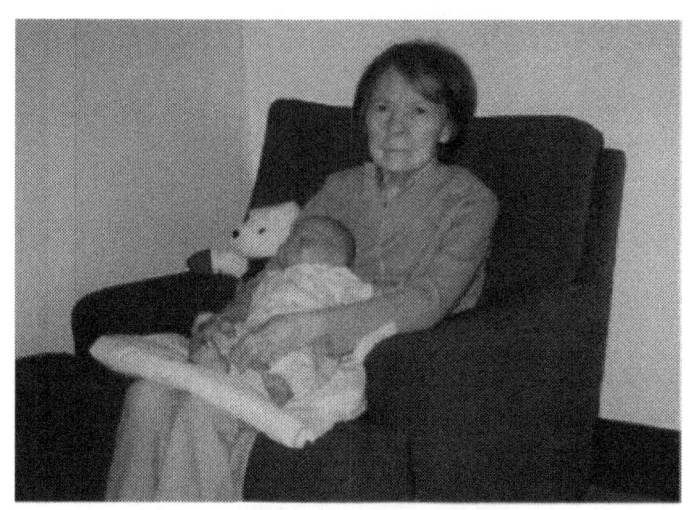

Wesley Gardens, 1994

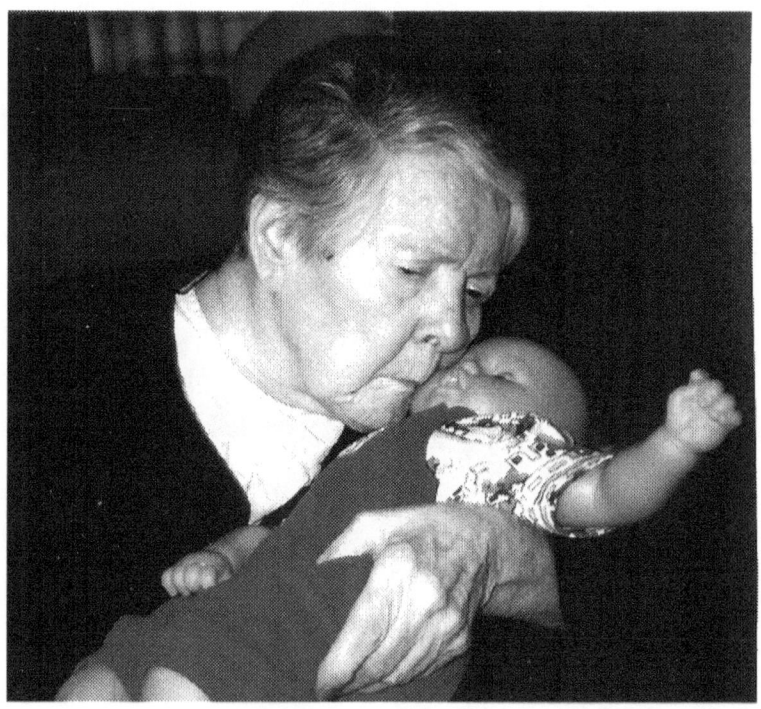

Wesley Gardens, 2000

CHAPTER 7

The caregivers

December 15, 1990

Last night Gary and I went out for a short while after dinner. Just as we were putting on our coats, Mom said, "You know, when I went out today, it was real windy. I went down the street and when I got as far as I was going and came back, the wind practically blew me home." After rather lengthy questioning yesterday and today, we pieced together that she got a notion to go out and find a store to buy some food. She went to the end of the block and when she didn't see a store, came back. She did admit tonight that it wasn't a real good idea. I think she kind of frightened herself, besides the fact that she got pretty cold. I told her we can't get to the store without driving. She seemed to accept that, but who knows. When she gets a notion in her head, she becomes driven to carry out whatever she's thinking. I had hoped we could put off getting day care till at least next fall, but maybe not.

Carole, I got your package and card. Thanks. I'll get the afghan wrapped for Mom. She'll love it I'm sure. Like I said, anything warm.

December 16, 1990

Well, I thought we had the Christmas thing all figured out. Yesterday, Mom asked me to take her to the store to buy some things. She wasn't sure for whom, but she said, "You're in touch with all those people. Who are they? Who will you buy presents for?" I told her I didn't buy for anyone except the people in this house and that she didn't have to either. So we went out to K-Mart and she started looking, aisle by aisle. I attempted to shorten the search a bit and suggested we look at paperback books. Surprise! Surprise! She agreed! Shortly thereafter, she had picked out four books for the four of us and didn't get bent out of shape over the price. So I thought that was settled. Later, at home, she brought out some jewelry; two necklaces and a pin that she wanted to give to someone. She asked me for the name of 'that girl' and I said Michelle. She said yes, that was the one, but who were the other two. So I decided to venture a guess and asked if she'd like to send these things to Carole, Susan and Virginia. She said "WHO?!" I repeated it and she said, "Virginia who?" I explained and she said no, they weren't the ones. I finally told her to give one to Michelle and keep the other two. On another day she said, "I'd like to get something for the girls. Oh, maybe not. I think they're all gone now – Mary, Helen and June." A couple times she had talked about buying gifts for the children, but when you ask her what children, she has no idea. Somewhere floating around in her mind is a vague memory of buying gifts for her sisters and brothers, later the four of us, and most recently, the grandchildren; but none of that is clear. She just knows there used to be several people to buy for. I don't want to tell her how many grand-children there are. She probably wouldn't believe me, and if she did, she'd have heart failure at the prospect of buying that many gifts.

December 21, 1990

Jacqui, we got your basket and absolutely loved it! I tried to spirit away the chocolate covered cherries before anyone saw them because I KNEW you had intended them just for me, but I got caught. We even managed to save some till Michelle got home last night.

Virginia, Mom got the sweatshirt you sent. Since it came in her name, she opened it right away instead of waiting till Christmas. She really likes it. I'm not sure she understood the printing on it, but she read it and found it funny anyway. She has put it under the tree so everyone can see it for a few days. She doesn't want to wear it till after Christmas.

I am so excited! I think I may have found someone to stay with Mom during the daytime. I have been concerned about which way to go with this, not wanting to go the home health aide route. The agencies won't necessarily send you the same person every day and it could get very confusing and disruptive for Mom to have different people here all the time.

A couple days ago, Gary was teaching at the police academy. A group was there during the morning doing role plays and they all went to lunch together. After lunch, as Gary was leaving, he kind of threw back over his shoulder, "Anybody want a job sitting for a woman with Alzheimer's?" Well, surprise, surprise! There was this woman there who had had occasion to do role plays for the academy now and then over the past few years so she and Gary have become somewhat acquainted. It turns out, she and a cousin of hers have taken care of a couple of Alzheimer's patients part time and the most recent one just died a week ago. She had been hoping to find a new position with some flexibility because she has a 4-yr-old son. She wanted an Alz. case, but wanted flexible hours and a place where she could bring her little boy. She was quite sure she'd never find a job to fit her needs. She said when Gary made that comment she was more than a little excited, because she had prayed for something to come along and here we were.

She and I talked this morning on the phone and she sounds really nice. She's very interested in staying with Mom, as is her cousin. She's going to call me in a few days and set up a time for the three of us to meet.

December 31, 1990

This is the last day I can write 1990. (Although I'm quite sure I'll forget to write 91 till at least March). Happy anniversary to Virginia & Bill and Susan & Charlie! Happy New Year!

I'm going to take our Christmas decorations down tomorrow, a little early for us – I usually wait till 'Little Christmas,' Jan. 6 – but for Mom's sake, we need to end this thing. We had to put all our gifts away the day after Christmas, because she couldn't stand to have all those things sitting under the tree. She spent all day Christmas sorting, stacking, reorganizing, opening and closing boxes, and eventually filtering things into her room.

The disarray made her crazy and her fussing around made Gary crazy. On Thursday, she wanted me to take her out shopping for Christmas cards to send. I couldn't convince her that she didn't have to and that Christmas was over, so I gave her a bunch I had and helped her address a few. (As you may have noticed, I didn't send any this year). She ended up taking them and tucking them away in her room so I don't know if she'll mail them or not. Christmas itself was odd to say the least. She had a bunch of stuff wrapped – treasures she had found around her room – and half of it she ended up giving to herself. Some of the things I knew she had wrapped a couple weeks earlier never appeared at all. The book she bought for David, she wrapped and gave to herself. The one she bought for Michelle, she gave to Gary and the other two never showed up. We bought her a winter coat and the kids got her a hat, scarf and gloves to go with it, but the next day, she insisted that the scarf and hat weren't hers. Yesterday a couple more wrapped items emerged from her room with strange notes on them like:

> Patty
> Have Drive to Bicitt
> a
> Comeononnon
> d

Now she's trying to figure out who to give them to. Thursday, Friday and Saturday she was up at the crack of dawn trying to get someone to take her to Church and Sunday she didn't realize we were actually going to Church until I got up and reminded her. I don't think I'll take her to Church tomorrow. It will be just one more disruption that she won't be able to digest. It's time we got her back on an even keel. The difficult part about it is that she ties all this excess confusion to Michelle. It all seemed to start when she appeared – must be her fault. Oh well, tomorrow we'll try to get back to normal again.

Meanwhile, on Saturday, I met with the two cousins who are going to be staying with Mom starting January 21, when Gary goes back to school. Their names are Debbie and Carolyn. They are the nicest people you could imagine. They are so enthused about doing this. We met for lunch and talked for over two hours. They've both cared for Alzheimer's patients and really enjoy older people. I told them all about Mom and what they could expect. They asked if they could take her out places and I assured them this would be a great idea. I'm hoping that if she gets used to having someone take her out fairly often, she'll stop greeting us at 6:00 and 7:00 a.m. with her coat and hat on. Debbie is going to come on Monday, Wednesday and Friday and Carolyn is going to be here on Tuesday and Thursday.

They're going to come over this Wednesday night to meet Mom and get familiar with the house and all. I'm not sure how Mom is going to take this, but she'll get used to it quickly enough I suppose. The two are so nice, it'll be impossible for her not to like them. I think she's getting a bit concerned about being alone lately anyway.

Virginia, Mom got your flowers (and Mrs. T. did too) and she loves them. Carole, we gave her the afghan on Christmas and she seemed to really be pleased with it. Of course, she has put it away in her room along with all her other gifts for now. She has a bit of difficulty breaking down and using something that's new. She likes to admire things for a while.

January 5, 1991

Debbie and Carolyn came over this past Wednesday to meet Mom and get a 2¢ tour of the house. Debbie asked if Mom had any idea why they were there and I said no, but I'd tell her before they left. Later, as they were getting their coats on, I told Mom that when Gary goes back to school, Debbie and Carolyn would be coming to stay with her during the day. They added they would be keeping her company and having lunch with her. She didn't seem to understand at first and then said, "Oh no, you can't make me . . . I have all this . . . and I can't . . ." It appeared that she thought they were going to be taking her away every day, so we explained they were coming here so she wouldn't be alone, whereupon she said, "Oh, well, that's all right." I think she'll find it disruptive at first, but she'll get used to it. I think this will be better than taking her out for day care. With that, I'd have to be sure she was up and dressed by a certain time every day and I have a feeling she'd fight going for quite a while. She's better off in a familiar place.

She seems rather more removed lately. Whether it's all because of the holidays or this is more progression (regression), I can't tell just yet. She wanted to make my bed this morning after I took off the sheets to wash them.

I got clean sheets out and she went off with them to make up the bed but kept coming back to ask what the pillow cases were for and how to put the sheets on, etc. When I take her out to the hairdresser or store, I have to tell her several times to put on her coat. She'll go in and out of her room, each time returning with something different on – a sweater, a spring jacket, a hat, boots – eventually finding the right coat. Right now it's 8:00 p.m. and she's downstairs waiting for someone to call and take her to Church. We've told her half a dozen times that Church is tomorrow, but she's still waiting, church envelope all ready.

January 13, 1991

Just as we expected, last Sunday, Mom was up by 4:00 a.m., coat and hat on, waiting to go to Church. She came up at 4:30, 5:00, 6:00 and 6:30 a.m. to ask when we were leaving. Gary got up shortly after that because he goes to Mass at 7:30 a.m. He told her over and over that our Mass is at 10:30 and each time she seemed satisfied with that answer for about ten minutes. By the time I came downstairs at a little after 10:00, she had given up hope of my ever taking her to Church, I guess, because she was fixing herself a sandwich. I told her she didn't have time to eat because we were going to Church and she said, "Well, then, I'm not going to Church!" I said that was fine and started to put my coat on. She panicked and ran for her coat and hat.

This week, she didn't come upstairs till after Gary left, but she did have her coat and hat on when he went out. She came up at about 8:30 a.m. and asked me if I was crazy. I felt like saying, "No more than usual," but I didn't. She said something about 'everybody on the street' and asked me to please get up. I told her Mass was at 10:30 and I would be up in time. She came back at 8:52. The reason I know it was 8:52 is because she said, "Patty! It's 8:52 and it says in the thing that all the Masses end at 8:52 so now won't you take me?" She has no real concept of time, but she can read a digital clock. I told her the Masses weren't all over, that we would go at 10:30 just like every other week and she was to go downstairs and wait till I told her it was time. I'm not sure why I kept telling her 10:30 because it doesn't mean a thing. She went away, seemingly satisfied and went to her room. 15 min. later, she was back. By now I had given up on sleeping and was reading a book. She said, "Patty, I . . .Patty, I . . .He said . . .He said . . .I think . . .well, he . . .I'm a Catholic you know." I said, "So am I. So what's your point?" (Stupid answer, I know). I went over the whole thing again and she went away one more time. Before she could appear again, I got up and went to take a shower and hung out in the bathroom for about half an hour. SO FAR, it's the one place she won't follow me.

Every morning this past week, she was up before dawn, coat and hat on, just waiting. Previously, she'd do that occasionally, thinking we were going to Church. When I'd tell her it wasn't Sunday, she'd be annoyed, but she'd take off her coat and give up. Lately, it's been happening almost every morning, and now, she just wants to go anywhere. Tuesdays, I take the garbage out in the morning before work, so I go out the back door. I came downstairs and there she was. I told her she wasn't going anywhere and she said, "Oh yes I am!" I told her, as usual, that it was dark out, no one was up, and nothing was open. As I put my jacket on, I said I was going to work and she said, "I'll go to work too." I told her she couldn't go out. I went out the back door and she stood there watching me. I locked the door with my key and as soon as I took the key out, she unlocked the door from the inside and opened it. I told her to stay inside. We went through this exercise again, and the third time, I attempted to lock the door, I had my key in the lock and my hand on the knob and she started pulling and yanking on the door for all she was worth. I had to stand there and hold the door shut till she calmed down and stopped. Fortunately, David was getting up about then. She finally gave up and walked away from the door, so I left. But after I drove out, I went around the block to see if she'd come out after I was out of sight. She didn't. David later said that she took her coat off before he left, but she didn't put it away. I think the saving grace these days is that it's been mighty cold and she hates the cold. One more week till Debbie and Carolyn start.

January 24, 1991

Week one of the 'Mom-sitters' and all is well. Monday, Gary stayed home till Debbie got here. She brought both her kids because the little girl (6-yr-old) didn't have school. Gary said Mom didn't object to his leaving, but later, when David got home around 2:00 p.m., he said she was acting weird. He said she didn't seem upset really, just weird. When he came in, she hugged and kissed him, which she never does. He went upstairs to do homework and Debbie stayed a while longer. He said Mom talked to the children, more clearly and understandably than she does to adults, and didn't seem to mind their being here. But she kept asking where Gary was. Debbie left about 3:00 p.m. and Gary came home shortly thereafter. By the time I got home, everything seemed normal. Actually, I thought Mom seemed calmer that evening, but then I realized that I was the one who was calmer.

Tuesday I stayed home till Carolyn got here about 9:00 a.m. Mom didn't seem to mind when I left. When I got home at 4:30, Carolyn said they had a pretty good day. She went to get her jacket to go home and Mom said, "Oh! You don't have to leave!" Carolyn assured her she would be back on Thursday and Mom said, "Well, I'll be here." Wednesday evening, Debbie called to see if I noticed any difference in Mom because she saw a big difference between Monday and Wednesday. She thought Wednesday went really well. Mom seemed much more accepting of her being there and really seemed to enjoy Danny. We think that on Monday, she was really thrown by having what she thought was company without our being there. Whether she was upset at having to entertain them alone or wondered if we were coming back at all, we're not sure, but she got over it. In fact, Wednesday through Friday, she wasn't up at 5:30 a.m. with her coat and hat on, waiting to go out. Of course, she was up again this morning, but she probably thought it was Sunday. She got her Church envelopes in the mail yesterday. But, hope springs eternal. I think this is going to work out well. When Debbie called she said, "This is just the kind of position I wanted. I am really enjoying being with your mother."

January 27, 1991

I wanted to get this out today, because I wanted to let you know that Uncle Jim died on Thursday. We just came back from the funeral home a little while ago. Cathy, (daughter-in-law) called Friday evening and told us about it. Apparently he died of heart failure while he was in Florida. I think his sister went over Thursday morning and found he had died during the night. He had told a couple of people that he had pains in his arm and shoulder for a few days previously, but when it was suggested he go to the doctor, he just brushed it off and said doctors only want to get your money.

We didn't take Mom to the funeral home. I doubt she would understand why we were there. She doesn't remember who Uncle Jim is anyway. Yesterday, she was all over the place. I guess being the end of the first week of 'Mom-sitters' and having Michelle home didn't help, and to top it off, there was a huge house fire three doors down from us last evening. She had been fussing and driving me crazy all afternoon. I finally took her out for a ride in the car to see if that would help to calm her. When we got back, about 15 minutes later, the street was blocked off. They let us down the street, but we had to park a few doors down because the fire hoses were across the driveway. All the commotion really put her out in left field. She didn't know we were home, and even after we were in the house for a while, she said the living room seemed smaller. Shortly thereafter, she said she had to go to the bathroom but she didn't know where it was. About an hour later, Michelle and I were going out to a color guard show and Mom begged and pleaded to come along. I kept telling her no, that it would be too long and too late and she pleaded some more and promised to behave the whole time – it was like trying to get away from a 3-yr-old. Later, Gary said he ended up taking her out for a ride again. Today she seemed a whole lot better, much more together, but she was quite surprised when we told her it was Sunday and we had to go to Church. There's just no predicting.

January 28, 1991

This morning, when I left for work, Mom was up and puttering around the kitchen, no coat, hat and boots. When I got home, Gary said he woke up at 7:45 a.m. to Mom standing over him staring into his face. She had the coat, hat and boots on then and wanted him to take her to Church. He said no, it wasn't Sunday and she went away. A few minutes later, he got up and went in to take a shower. The next thing he knew, there was a firm knocking on the bathroom door. He opened it to find the guy from next door standing there. Mom had waited till Gary got in the shower and went next door to get someone to take her to Church.

Gary had to go to school, so David stayed around till Debbie showed up. When she got here, Mom was standing by the front window saying, "I'm going to get out of here." So Debbie said, "Come on; you and I will go for a little ride." Later in the day, when Debbie was getting ready to go home, Mom didn't want her to leave, so Debbie said maybe Carolyn would take her out tomorrow. Mom said, "Who's Carolyn?"

When I got home, Mom seemed fine, but just a little while ago (it's 9:20 p.m.) she got up and headed for her room. We assumed she was going to bed. Ten minutes later, she was back, dressed to go out. Gary and David had to do plenty of talking to get her away from the door. I think tomorrow I'll have to return to our plan of getting two-way locks. We'll have them put on right above the current locks so we only have to use the double locks at night (or when we're in the shower, I guess). With Debbie and Carolyn coming now, there won't be much time that she's alone. Actually the time we'll need the double locks (other than at night) is from the time I go to work until Gary or David get up.

January 29, 1991

Well, we now have double keyed locks on all the doors. I had one put on the door going outside from her room even though she has never opened it, because she just might try it one day. It's odd that she doesn't seem to be aware that she could open that door and head outside with no one noticing, but it's as if she doesn't even know it's there. She never even had it open in the summer.

I had keys made for the four of us, for Debbie and Carolyn and for the people next door. Now the major decision is, do we lock the doors on Tuesday and Thursday mornings from the time Gary goes to school till Carolyn gets here. If we do, we're taking a big risk; if we don't, she may take off and be long gone before Carolyn gets here. We'll see.

CHAPTER 8

More adventures in caregiving and an ice storm

February 1, 1991

We decided not to use the locks on Tuesday and Thursday mornings. Hopefully, the cold weather will deter her and our next door neighbor said she'd keep an eye out for her.

Debbie called me Wednesday night to let me know that Mom had a fit when she (Debbie) was leaving that day. She wanted to call because she thought it upset David and she figured when David told me about it, I'd be concerned that it upset Debbie too. She wanted to assure me that it didn't. Apparently this happened on Monday too. Mom was fine all while Debbie was here, but when it was time for her to leave, Mom got all agitated and angry. We aren't sure whether she was upset because Debbie was leaving or because she wasn't taking Mom with her or because Gary and I weren't home yet. David said you couldn't make any sense out of what she was saying. He went downstairs to prevent her from following Debbie out the door and he said the last thing she said as Debbie closed the door behind her was "Oh! You!" and made a motion like she was going to kick her. Fortunately, Debbie didn't see that. This afternoon, David said she slipped out while Mom was upstairs making beds and Mom made no comment later when she realized Debbie was gone.

I made the mistake of telling Mom last night that Debbie was going to take her to the store today. She fluttered all around for the next hour and finally went to bed around 9:00 p.m. She was back up at about 11:00 p.m. with her coat, hat and boots on and wouldn't listen to Gary at all when he told her to go back to bed. So he gave up and let her sit there while he watched TV. He was coming to bed at 1:00 a.m. and it took some doing to convince her that she couldn't stay up. She finally went in to bed, but was up again around 5:00 a.m. When I came down at 6:00, she was just sitting on the couch, in the dark, hat, coat and boots on, waiting. Presumably, she went on waiting till Debbie showed up at 9:30.

February 8, 1991

Thought I had a golden opportunity today, but I just missed it. Debbie called me at work to let me know she had to take her daughter for a doctor's appointment. She was going to take Mom along, then go to her house for lunch and make cookies in the afternoon. She wanted me to know that if I got home from work and Mom wasn't around, not to worry. After I hung up, I asked my boss if I could leave work an hour early or so to take advantage of a quiet, empty house. He said fine, so I left at 3:30, stopped at the post office for the mail and got home about 3:45. Guess who rolled in around 3:50? Oh well, just my luck.

Michelle is home again this weekend. Actually she sort of passed through on her way to a party in Buffalo. I'm quite sure it was her though.

Gary's gone on a bus trip to a Sabres game in Buffalo and David is either with him or at a hockey game at RIT. Tomorrow Gary is supposed to be going on a ski trip to someplace near the Adirondacks, but it's been around 50 degrees here all week and not a bit of snow is left. I doubt the place he's going will have much either. It was supposedly warm all over the state all week. Maybe he can go mud skiing or something.

February 11, 1991

Every now and then when I think things are finally going smoothly, I get dragged back to reality. This past weekend went by reasonably; no major upsets. This morning, one of the people at work was asking how the 'Mom-sitters' were working out and I was saying that it was really great. She seems to like them and they like her and they take her out fairly often. Debbie hadn't said anything about problems when she was leaving this past week.

The double keyed locks keep Mom inside when we're sleeping (or showering). Everything was going fine. Then about 2:30 p.m., Debbie called me at work sounding rather frantic. She was getting ready to leave to pick up her daughter from school and Mom decided to have a fit. Neither David nor Gary was home yet. Debbie tried to calm her down, but Mom went and put on her coat and boots, dashed outside, got into the driver's side of Debbie's car and refused to get out. She would scream every time Debbie tried to talk to her. I told her to tell Mom that I would be home soon and that she had to be home when I got there. If that didn't get her back in the house, I'd come right home. Debbie said okay, and if I didn't hear from her within about ten minutes, I could assume that it worked. About five minutes later, our secretary came in my office and asked if Mom knew how to call me at work. I said yes (she has the lab phone number on the refrigerator) and she said, "Well, I think she's on the phone. I can't understand her." Sure enough, it was Mom ranting and raving and making very little sense. I tried to tell her that Debbie had to go to pick up her daughter at school, but that was futile. Nothing I said made sense to her. In fact, at one point, she decided it wasn't me on the phone. I told her to sit down and watch television and, suddenly, I thought she hung up on me, but then David got on the phone. Fortunately, he came in just as Debbie was getting Mom back in the house. She quickly explained what was happening and asked him to call me. He went upstairs to take his coat off and Mom got to the phone first. He said Mom wasn't making any sense and he didn't know what, if anything, he could do for her. I told him that was okay. All he had to do was keep her from leaving.

When Gary got home, I told him the story and he said he would make a concerted effort to get home by 2:30 from now on.

I just talked to Debbie on the phone. This whole episode really shook her. After we talked for a while, I said I hoped it wouldn't scare her off. She said it would take more than that. She said Mom was somewhat tense and agitated all day, and being left alone apparently didn't set too well. She said when she got off the phone after talking to me, she went outside. Mom was out of the car and trying to get Danny out of the back seat. Debbie told her what I had said and finally got her to go back in the house. David walked in to find Debbie shaking like a leaf and crying, and Mom pacing and angry. Lucky David.

February 17, 1991

This upcoming week is winter break for the schools around here. Coincidentally, Carolyn and her husband are on vacation. Originally, before they started coming, Carolyn and Debbie asked what I wanted to do about this week and I said it was no problem because Gary is off too. As things progressed, Debbie suggested that she would come on her days anyway to kind of keep Mom to a routine. The week before last, she had both kids with her because her daughter was out of school with a cough. Things went pretty well, so she decided it would work out okay to come this week and give Gary a chance to go skiing or whatever.

Then Friday she called and said this past week had been emotionally draining and the kids were real rambunctious and that might be pretty stressful for Mom. Bottom line was, she was asking if I minded if she didn't come after all. In fact, I don't mind, because Gary is off, and we had originally agreed to this. What concerns me is that I'm beginning to get the impression that Debbie came into this situation with the idea, or hope, that she could somehow make Mom better. She really likes Mom and says she enjoys being with her, but I don't want to have to add Debbie to the list of people whose well-being I have to worry about. Hopefully, a week's break will do her good.

February 24, 1991

A week without 'Mom-sitters' and Gary is ready to go back to school. It should be interesting to see how the day goes when Debbie and Danny come back tomorrow. Debbie called on Wednesday to see how Mom was and let us know she was thinking about us. (She's so kind). She asked if the disruption in routine had an effect on her, and I told her I didn't look at it all that closely. Mom has good days and bad days and I just try to deal with them as they come.

February 27, 1991

Debbie and Carolyn's return doesn't seem to have made a difference, although yesterday Mom did try to get Carolyn to spend the night.

I've had two phone calls from Susan in the past few days. One was to say her company set her up with an office at home and an 800 phone number. I'm so jealous! Imagine being able to roll out of bed and stumble to your desk without having to fully wake up and go out somewhere. Sounds really inviting! The other call was to see if we want to meet her and Charlie in Philadelphia the weekend of April 19-21. She's got a Mary Kay thing going on. Charlie had suggested that Gary go down to play golf with him while Susan is at her meetings and Susan figured it would be a good idea if I came along since her meetings won't be taking up the whole weekend. I told her I'd see.

March 4, 1991

It's about 11:30 a.m. It seems like it should be at least dinner time. I've been up since 5:30 a.m. and I'm not at work because we had this huge ice storm during the night. I got up at the regular time to go to work and, in spite of the fact that the radio was announcing all sorts of school closings, I was sure I could get to work. After all, it's only ten minutes away. I went out into an absolutely transformed street. It was so pretty and, as I soon discovered, so dangerous. The driveway and street weren't icy, but after 20 minutes of scraping the ice off my car, I walked out into the street to move a branch out of my way, I looked up and down the street and saw huge limbs down everywhere. There was no getting out. Besides which, every few seconds, you'd hear a loud crack and more limbs would fall like thunder. When they hit the ground, it was like the sound of dozens of glasses breaking as the ice flew in every direction. I still attempted to get out, weaving around branches but was totally blocked about five houses away. So I turned around and came home. I ran up and woke Gary and told him to grab his camera and come outside with me. We went out with two cameras and wandered up and down the street taking pictures; it was just so unbelievable. By that time, (about 7:00 a.m.) people were everywhere with cameras and videos, filming and dodging, filming and dodging. When I called in to work, only one guy had gotten there and was sorry he did because he wasn't looking forward to trying to get back home again.

Now the branches are just falling occasionally, but the rain has turned to snow and it's a heavy wet snow. The TV people are warning everyone to stay inside because more branches and power lines are going to come down as the day goes on. In fact, it's amazing that I'm able to write you. We're among a very few people who have power. But we're being warned that it may not last. Mom is just taken with how pretty everything looks. The tree out back has some red buds on it and the branches that haven't fallen off are drooped to the ground with ice. So the view from her window is very picturesque. I'm surprised she hasn't had any interest in going outside, because we've made three trips out with cameras, going a little farther each time, but she doesn't seem to mind our leaving her inside alone. She seems more fascinated than afraid.

Michelle came home from school last night. She got in about midnight and said branches were starting to fall as she neared the Rochester area. I wasn't aware of it till two or three in the morning. Now Mom is really convinced that Michelle brings disaster. First there was the confusion of Christmas, and then there was that house fire down the street. This time, she's managed to damage the whole street.

The last trip we made outside, Gary went farther than I did and said he saw some car damage on the streets a few blocks from us. On the TV, they showed a street where a power line was down at an angle across a road and car after car was driving under it. Here on our street, I saw two teenage girls with a little kid about 3 or 4 years old. The girls were going up on the lawns and looking at damaged bushes and trees down in backyards and the little boy was dancing around in the street when a branch came crashing down not 5 feet from him. The girls turned around when they heard it, but then went on about their business with no more regard for the child than they had before. Makes you wonder.

Ed[1] called a while ago and said their mother has power at her apartment. I thought of her earlier today, but we couldn't get out to get her if we wanted to. He said they lost power out their way and tried to get out this morning to get breakfast, but were stopped by the police and told to go back home. They live in a housing tract that isn't old enough to have any big trees so they didn't realize what it was like when they set out.

Two days ago, it was 68 degrees and sunny and I had the house open all day and cleaned out the front garden.

---

[1] Ed and Sue are Gary's brother and sister-in-law.

March 5, 1991

Jim & Sandy came over for dinner last night because they're without power and heat. There are over 250,000 homes without power in the area. They say they won't be restored for four to seven days. There are shelters set up at several schools including Monroe Community College. Gary thought he'd be going to school today, but he'd have a hard time stepping over all those people.

Another day home; another day of taking pictures. These should be even better than yesterday's because the sun is shining. The iced-over trees look spectacular. My boss called last night and said the company would be closed today. About the only things open were Kodak and a few stores. Only 6 of the 24 Wegmans stores had power. By late morning, the sun was starting to melt the ice off the trees and it was coming down in showers. About 3:00 p.m., I went out to start cleaning up the yard as best I could. We now have a HUGE pile of branches and limbs out by the curb as does everyone else. While I was out, there were people all up and down the street using chain saws and dragging branches around. A gas and electric crew came through last night about 11:00 p.m. with a front-loader and cleared all the branches out of the street, but first thing this morning, we heard on the radio that police were ticketing people who went out in their cars without an extremely good reason.

Now the streets and yards look horrid. The ice is all melted and everything is a mess. The trees look so pitiful. The newspaper estimated that 90% of the county's trees have been damaged but we won't know just how badly until spring and summer. One reporter wrote ". . .but no one will be able to tell there was tree damage ten years from now." Somehow that's not encouraging.

Gary was appointed the task of getting a key for the upstairs bathroom door today, but he hasn't done it yet. I've been trying to keep Mom out of our bathroom, but with no success. Then on Sunday, David caught her cleaning the sink and counter with my washcloth. (Mind you, she doesn't do this in her bathroom). The next day, he found her cleaning the sink with garbage from the wastebasket. He stopped her and as soon as he walked away, she did it again; so he stopped her again. She closed the door on him and he heard the toilet flush twice. When she came out, he went in to check and, sure enough, she had clogged the toilet trying to flush the garbage down it. So now, until Gary gets a lock on the door, we have to hide our washcloths and not put anything in the wastebasket. But I know she'll find something else to get into.

March 6, 1991

Back to work today, and was Mom ever thrilled! When I got up to leave this morning, I found her waiting in the dark with coat, hat and boots which is nothing new. The new angle was that she was hell-bent on going with me. Usually when I tell her I have to go to work, she grumbles and complains, but stays in. This time, she planted herself in front of the door shouting, "I AM going!" I took her by the arm and pulled her back into the living room and told her she couldn't come whereupon she hauled off and smacked me with her purse and then did it a second time. I told her to stop that and stay inside. As I tried to open the door, she grabbed the edge of the door and tried to squeeze past me. I took her by both arms and maneuvered her back inside again which prompted her to punch me with her fist. It was barely more than a thump, given her whopping 90 pounds or so, but she put everything she had into it. I managed to slip out and get the door locked. I could hear her pounding on it as I walked down the driveway.

Later, Michelle told me that she pounded on the door for a minute or so, then came upstairs and hollered at Gary about how mean I was and insisted that he get up and take her out NOW! He told her to go away. She did, but then went down and banged on the front and back doors for a bit and finally came back upstairs and stood in our room watching and waiting. She didn't say anything more, but stood for about half an hour waiting for Gary. He kept telling her to go away, and that, after all, he doesn't watch her sleeping. Later, when Michelle got up, Mom told her how mean I was and how I kicked her, punched her and knocked her down. Oh well. . .

We went out to dinner for her birthday tonight and everything's back to 'normal.' I just can't wait for tomorrow morning!

March 8, 1991

Yesterday morning, Mom was still sleeping when I left for work – highly unusual. She must have worn herself out or maybe it was my 'beating her up' that did it. This morning I could hear her up and waiting when I woke up. By the time I was ready to go downstairs, she was in the kitchen. She had her back to the front door and was furtively wolfing down cake out of the pan with her hands. By some miracle of chance, I was able to get my jacket on and slip out without her hearing me.

Carolyn came today because Debbie is still without power in her house. She said when she came in, Mom was all annoyed and saying that she wasn't going to talk to anyone again. She took Carolyn in the kitchen and showed her a bag of donuts that Gary had bought earlier. She took each one out saying, "Look at this! Nothing in it!" Apparently she wanted filled donuts. She calmed down as the day went on and was fine by the time I got home.

March 17, 1991

Happy St. Patrick's Day! Too bad I can't print this in green.

On Friday, about 9:20 a.m. I got a call at work. When I answered the phone, I heard Debbie's voice on the verge of panic saying, "Where's your mother?!" She proceeded to tell me that she had just arrived and Mom was nowhere in the house, but her purse and gloves were on the counter in the kitchen. Gary wasn't around and the front door wasn't locked. Then she said to wait, that she'd go back to Mom's room. Perhaps Mom had fallen and Debbie didn't see her at first. As she left the phone, I heard Gary's voice in the background saying "Hi! I'll bet you were wondering where we were, huh?" Apparently he had taken her out to the store. Debbie came back to the phone and said she'd strangle Gary after she hung up. I agreed that was an appropriate plan and hung up. Set me on edge for the rest of the morning.

Last weekend, Mom was just aching to get outside all morning (that is, from about 5:00a.m. on). Finally, when I got up and unlocked the doors, she fled out the door to go clean up the front lawn. I told her she couldn't rake because it was too early in the season for that, but she could pick up sticks and branches left from the ice storm. She was satisfied with that since that was what was making her crazy anyway – looking at all those sticks from the front window. She ended up spending about two hours outside picking up every little thing on the lawn. She finally came in complaining of being stiff and sore, but about half an hour later, she was back at it again. I thought for sure she'd be a wreck the next day, but she wasn't. In fact, Sunday morning she came and woke me up at 8:30 with her work clothes on asking if I'd unlock the door so she could go back out. She got genuinely annoyed when I told her it was Sunday and we had to go to Church. I thought she'd head out right after Church, but she didn't. Monday, it was cold and rainy, so her project got delayed till Tuesday. Carolyn told me she spent about another two hours out there that day too. I had told Carolyn to let her rake or sweep or whatever when the weather was nice. Mom enjoys it and she's much calmer in the evening when she's been out.

March 23, 1991

Debbie called me last night to sort of check in. I had seen her earlier this week although I don't usually. On Monday, she called me at work about 9:30 a.m. to say she was at our next door neighbor's because she had forgotten her key. I said something about the fact that I have asked Gary not to double lock the door when he goes out, but she said she hadn't checked that. She figured if she knocked on the door and Mom couldn't get it open, she would be very upset. Our one neighbor who has a set of keys wasn't home, so Debbie came over to work and got my keys.

Anyway, back to her call last night; she and I chatted about Mom for a bit. She said she feels like she's gotten over her earlier apprehension and really loves coming to stay with Mom now. She doesn't know what she'll do when the day comes that I need more 'professional' help to take care of Mom. "I really love this job." I was very pleased and relieved to hear her say that.

Gary's in Boston this weekend. He managed to get tickets to see the Sabres play the Bruins. One of his hockey buddies went along too. Too bad Buffalo lost today. David watched part of the game on TV and said they didn't play very well. Oh well, Gary likes hockey no matter who wins.

March 29, 1991

Sure enough, Gary did enjoy the game in spite of the Sabres losing. They had a good weekend; however, it could have been better. They had thunder storms just like we did here, so they didn't get to do any walking around while they were there. It was too bad because the guy who went along had never been to Boston before.

I had off from work today. Debbie had called earlier in the week and offered to come and take Mom to her house for lunch so I could have time to myself. (Bless her!) I didn't hesitate to take her up on the offer. She picked Mom up at 11:00 a.m. and brought her back at 3:30 p.m. I didn't do much; just hung out and enjoyed the peace and absence of a shadow. I ran a few errands, cleaned Mom's bathroom, and fixed and ate lunch all by myself. By the time the afternoon was over, I was mentally prepared to have a pleasant evening. We'd watch some TV, have dinner, and I'd take her to Church for Stations of the Cross (every Friday during Lent). Sounded good.

When they got home, as they got out of the car, the kids wanted to walk down the street. Debbie told them they could, but stay on the sidewalk and only go two houses down. Mom jumped out of the car and started hollering at them, "You two stay right in this yard! Get back here now!" Debbie was saying, "Bea, it's okay. Bea! I told them they could go. They'll be fine. Let's go in the house." All the while, she had to physically direct her to the door as Mom protested vehemently. She finally came in and hurried over to the front window to watch. By this time, the kids were picking up a few stray branches and tossing them up on the roadside piles. Mom was frantic. "Look at that! Look at that! We have to stop them! Now they can't. . ." and the rest became unintelligible. Debbie was standing in the front doorway and I was between her and Mom when Mom made a dash for the door, thoroughly put out that Debbie was doing nothing to stop those kids. She was muttering, "Well, I'll just. . ." when I stopped her in her tracks. She fought to get away, but I got her attention and said, "They're not your kids! They're Debbie's and she will take care of them." Just then, Amanda came in and Debbie said goodbye and hurried out the door. Mom watched out the window as they left and apparently saw Amanda get in the car but didn't see Danny. She said, "Where's the little boy?" and as they backed out, "Oh, he's in the car already." and that was the end of that, or so I thought.

A short time later, she was upstairs in my bathroom and I had to go chase her out. After that, she seemed restless, pacing back and forth and looking out the front window. Gary had come home and we were just watching TV and reading the paper. Finally she went into her room for a bit, came back out and went out the back door. I thought she was going out in the yard as she often does, but as I watched, I saw her come around the house and head down the sidewalk. I went out and caught up with her a couple doors down. I asked her where she was going and she said, "I have to go there cause he. . ." and the rest made no sense. I told her she didn't have to go anywhere. She turned and followed me home without hesitation. Then she spent another half hour pacing and wringing her hands and practically knocking over my plants in order to see out the front window. She would sit down and get up and sit down and get up and then she started this loud sighing and these hesitant little noises like she was going to say something, but she didn't. It was making my hair stand on end. Finally, on the verge of tears, she asked me something about "those little kids" and I managed to figure out that she thought Danny had gone down the street and was probably lost. That's where she was headed when she went out. I assured her that they had gone home and that Danny was in the car when they left. She seemed immensely relieved, but about 20 minutes later she started asking about him again. It was as if she suddenly remember that she was supposed to be worried about something, but then again, maybe not. I told her again the kids were home and fine and she finally dropped it.

We had a major windstorm Thursday. Signs and streetlights blew down, some large windows blew out and a whole lot of fir trees were totally uprooted. There was a beautiful one right across the street from us that just fell right over. That was the one kind of tree that wasn't damaged by the ice storm because the branches hang downward anyway, but they must have been weakened by the storm because there were lots of them down yesterday. About 12,000 homes lost power again. I wonder what April will be like.

CHAPTER 9

Exhaustion

April 14, 1991

It's been quite a while since I wrote. It seems I've come to the end of my rope and I've found the end extremely frayed. In the past week I've felt about 30 seconds this side of a nervous breakdown. This whole situation with Mom will be coming to an end soon. It's beginning to affect my health, both mental and physical, my job and the family. I can't do it any more.

Up until last Saturday, I spent every waking moment worrying about her. Even though we got the double keyed locks, I still wake up at night when she gets up – 1:00 a.m., 3:00 a.m., 4:00 a.m., whatever. After I get up at 5:30 and shower, I have to hide my washcloth so she won't clean the bathroom with it during the day (just mine, it turns out – she doesn't use any one else's). I have to remember to turn off the phone which cuts me off from contacting Debbie or Carolyn. Then I have to sneak out without eating breakfast in hopes of avoiding a conflict to start the day off. Sometimes I make it, sometimes I don't. Then from about 6:30 to 9:30 a.m., I spend the time worrying whether she has gotten out of the house and wandered off, or wakened the neighbors. Or has Gary forgotten to unlock the doors and is she setting the house on fire. From about 9:15 to 9:45 a.m., if my phone rings, I about jump out of my skin because I'm sure it's Debbie calling to report a problem. Then I get about 5 hours of semi-peace till about 2:15 p.m. when the process reverses itself. I dread leaving work in the evening and can rarely ever work late unless I've arranged beforehand with Gary.

Once home, Mom's right on my heels. She wants to go out all the time, and if we go out, in very short order, she wants to go home. She snarls and complains about Gary most of the time which really bothers me since he has done nothing but try to help out. The only time she's nice to him is if she's mad at me; then she's overly sweet to him. Trying to talk to her is another whole issue. It's like trying to communicate with someone who neither speaks nor understands English. I rarely can make heads or tails out of what she is saying and when I talk to her, I get past three words and she's lost. Even simple things like, "Go get your coat." She'll say okay and just stand there and look at you. About the third time around, she'll go into her room, spend a great deal of time and come out without it.

And this is just the tip of the iceberg. It doesn't begin to cover the picture from Gary and David's points of view. Gary can't stay at school on Monday, Wednesday or Friday because he has to get home so Mom doesn't hassle Debbie. When David is the one to relieve Debbie, he doesn't know what to do when Mom cries or has fits. Gary and I can't just go out on the spur of the moment, and travel is out of the question. Gary and David get away, and I want them to, but we can't go anywhere together. They get to see Michelle periodically, but I can't unless she comes here. When she's here, that's never completely enjoyable anymore because Mom sees her as an intruder. She gives Michelle – and her friends – a hard time. Her friends come around less and less often.

And this Easter, Michelle didn't come home at all.

So now we come to last Sunday. Gary and David had gone out to a hockey game. It was a beautiful day and I had been outside a good part of the afternoon washing my car. For some reason, Mom never stepped out the door all day long. About 7:00 p.m. she decided it would be a good time to rake the lawn. She had been raking the front lawn constantly for the past couple of weeks and Gary asked me to stop her because she was raking the grass out by its roots. It was still light out, so I said if she wanted to rake, to rake the back yard; the front didn't need it. She glared at me, marched out the door, got the rake and went out front. I went out the front door and said, "I asked you not to do that." She looked up at me, scowled and went back to raking. So I went over and took hold of the rake and said, "If you want to rake, rake the back yard." Well, she started yanking and pulling on the rake, all the while trying to kick me and bite my hands. The whole thing went downhill from there. I finally had to give up or bodily carry her in the house kicking and yelling. I figured the neighbors had already seen enough, so I went back inside and slammed the door till it practically turned inside out.

With that, something just sort of snapped inside my head. What followed throughout this past week was a massive case of nerves which I still haven't been able to get under control. My stomach is upset when I wake up in the morning, headaches come and go through the day, I have heartburn, I can't concentrate at work, I've been on the verge of tears if I talk to anyone, and things aren't improving. Friday, I had planned to take the day off and go shopping with Sandy and some of her friends from work. We had the date set for some time. I went over to her house early and told her what was going on and she said she would help any way she could. We were going to go to Niagara Falls shopping and I thought I was doing pretty well that morning after we talked and her friends showed up. But as we drove, I started feeling sick and got worse and worse as we went along. I assumed it was just tension and motion sickness and I'd be fine when we got there, but I didn't feel any better once we got to where we were going. I felt terrible at the prospect of ruining Sandy's day off, and even if she were to take me all the way back, I wouldn't want to go home, so I had her take me to a motel nearby. I assured her this was exactly what I needed and that she was to go enjoy herself. So it worked out. I slept about four hours and then just watched some TV for another two. I still felt a little rocky when she got back, but the afternoon was extremely relaxing. When we got back to town, I stayed at Jim & Sandy's for a while and we talked about what's next. Sandy offered to go with me to check out some nursing homes. I had already talked to Gary and David about it on Wednesday. I asked Gary what he thought about Mom moving to a nursing home and he said he thought it was time about four months ago when we had to start day care and put double keyed locks on the doors, but he didn't feel it was his place to say so. Later when I asked David, he basically said it wasn't his or Gary's decision; it was mine and I had to be the one to make it.

The thing is, I know it's going to get worse before it gets better. I have this picture of what things will be like down the road when she's settled in someplace and I can go to see her and take her out at my discretion. It's the only way I can see clearly to getting back to some semblance of a reasonable relationship with her. During this past week, I've been aware of this whole part of my brain just shutting down – the part that has been worrying 24 hours a day. I've reached the point where I don't or can't care any more. I just want her out. Definitely not a beneficial attitude, I know, but that's the way it is. Tomorrow I'm going to put the wheels in motion and let the chips fall where they may. I have no idea how I'm going to tell her, but I can't think about that now. Today, we had another major fight about her 'cleaning' my bathroom with my washcloth, which I forgot to hide, and I nearly told her then, except that Gary interceded and warded off disaster.

So there it is. By the time you read this letter, I will have already started on the road to getting my life back on track. Hopefully I won't lose my sanity in the process.

CHAPTER 10

Nursing home placement

May 29, 1991

I should begin with a catch up of events for Aunt June since last I wrote, for Virginia and Carole since three weeks ago and for Susan since the day before yesterday.

As you recall back in mid-April, I was on the verge of a nervous breakdown. Well, I decided not to have one after all since it seemed like too much trouble. I did, however, go to my doctor the following week to see if I was going to be sick for the rest of my life and/or have a heart attack. He said all of my physical symptoms were stress related and gave me mild tranquilizers. I have only had occasion to use them twice (which is a milestone in and of itself since I don't take medicines), but I carry them in my purse as a security blanket sort of thing.

The Wednesday after I wrote, I had a nurse come over to do a 'PRI' evaluation, which is a 'Patient Review Instrument' that health care facilities need to see before they'll talk to you about placement. It only took about half an hour and Mom seemed to like the girl who did it. She was very happy to talk to her. Later that week, Sandy and I started making appointments to see a few nursing homes around town. I was going on the references of friends at work. By the weekend, I had decided if my impression of the place we were to see on Monday was the same as all the others, I would just start sending in applications.

As luck would have it, we went to see a place on Monday called Wesley on East, which is a complex on East Avenue and Goodman Street. It has four different facilities ranging from independent apartment living to skilled nursing care. We went to see the 'health related facility' called Upton Court. We were very impressed. On the main floor, it has a large living area, beautifully decorated, and a common dining room which looks like a restaurant. The basement floor has a laundry room which the residents or their families or the staff can use, a little sundry store, a craft room, a whirlpool, a hairdresser and a large activity hall. The residents' rooms are on the 2nd to 7th floors and each floor has a lounge area and a kitchenette. The rooms are quite good sized and carpeted and the residents can lock them if they want to. (The staff has keys, of course). The residents bring their own furniture, including their own bed. There's a little chapel on the main floor and they have a Catholic Mass or Communion service on Sundays, although it's a Methodist facility.

The intake social worker we met with that day said we needed to submit an application, the PRI and then they would contact Mom's doctor for medical information. If all that is in order, they have Mom in for an interview and assessment. She also said if, at that point, everything checks out, it wouldn't be any time at all till she could move in.

I went home that day and filled out and sent in the application and had the nurse who had done the PRI send a copy to Wesley. By the following Monday, I hadn't heard anything so I called and was told the PRI hadn't arrived yet. She said she would contact the doctor that day and I called again for the PRI. The woman hand delivered it that afternoon.

The following weekend, May 4/5, much to my surprise and delight and amazement, Susan and Virginia and Carole showed up on my doorstep. Actually, they showed up in a restaurant at which point I'd have fallen off my seat in shock except that I was sitting in the back of a booth and had nowhere to fall. We had a terrific weekend, hung out and drove around town most of the day Saturday and took in a comedy club that evening. On Sunday, Virginia and Carole had a late afternoon flight back to Phoenix, so we went out to lunch at the mall. Those two days were a great morale booster which has carried me through these last three weeks. Mom didn't seem to know them when she first saw them on Saturday, but after spending the whole day together, we believe she did know them by Sunday.

June 5, 1991

Time does get by me. I have to catch up in a hurry here because things have happened rather rapidly in the last few days.

The Monday after our 'reunion' weekend, I called the doctor's office and found out that they hadn't done anything about the medical report because they never got a final report from Monroe Community Hospital for Mom's geriatric assessment back in November of 1989. So I called over there and talked to someone who kept insisting that according to their files, I never came back for the final closure appointment. I kept insisting that I had been there and gave her the date and names of the people I talked to, but somehow they lost the final report and since it never made its way to Mom's file, obviously I was never there. There was no convincing her, so I got back to the doctor's office and set up an appointment for Mom to have another physical the following Friday which was all right because she was due anyway, but it held things up by another week. Then after the physical, we had to wait another week to get the blood work back before a report could go out to Wesley.

Another respite weekend – Memorial Day – Susan and Charlie came up for David's graduation. We had a really good time. Susan and Charlie got to spend a fun afternoon with Mom while Gary, Michelle and I went to the graduation Saturday. Mom went out to watch Charlie wash the cars and little by little started gathering sticks and grass and stuff from the lawn, driveway, sidewalk, street, etc. Soon, she had little piles of debris all around and wanted Charlie to help her clean them up. I guess he assumed it would wait till he was done with the cars. He should have known better. After a bit, Mom went in the house and came back out with her white jacket ready to scoop up the sticks with it. Charlie discovered that Mom doesn't understand the concept of 'later.' As he was sweeping the stuff up, our next door neighbor came by and said, "I see Grandma's got you working, huh?" She's well known on the street. Later, Charlie had gone out in the car and Mom was getting restless so Susan asked her if she'd like to go for a walk. Well, somewhere along the way, Mom decided Susan was looking for Charlie, so she tried to go up to each house and ask if he was there. Susan kept telling her there was no one home at that house. . .or that one. . .or that one. . .etc.

Anyway, the following Wednesday, I finally got an appointment to take Mom into Wesley on East for her evaluation. She went along willingly and was quite happy to talk to the social worker and nurse we met that day. However, in the course of the conversation, the nurse indicated that she didn't feel that they would have the appropriate amount of supervision for Mom. The doors are always unlocked from the inside. After 9:00 p.m. there's no one at the front desk and there's never anyone watching the back door. Basically, she was saying that if someone wanted to walk out, it would be relatively easy to do without being discovered.

I left the interview feeling discouraged because Upton Court was so nice. They said Goodman Gardens had better security, but it's a skilled nursing facility and perhaps not appropriate for her needs. The next day, I called to have copies of the PRI sent to four other nursing homes. I was told to call each place and let them know the form was coming. The first place I called is about ten minutes from where I work. The woman I spoke to said she was delighted I had called because a vacancy was just about to come up in a double room and I could come over and see it that same day. I went over about 3:30 that afternoon and took a look around. They have this unit which is specifically for people with Alzheimer's or other types of dementia, but who are still physically able to function. My initial reaction was not great because this place is definitely one with a nursing home/hospital appearance, and the room, as I said, is a double. People can decorate their rooms however they like and some that I saw were very homey and warm looking. I told the social worker about Wesley and why I was hesitant, and she said she certainly understood. She said she needed an answer by Monday about this room, but if I needed more time, Mom would certainly be put on a waiting list for the next room with no problem. Over the weekend, I talked to several people – Jim & Sandy, Carolyn, Debbie and Marcy. Marcy used to work at St. John's Home and I wanted to get some information about that place too. She called me back a couple days later and said she checked with a couple of people and found out that Mom would probably fall through the cracks there too; not enough supervision in the health related facility and too much in the skilled nursing facility.

June 7, 1991

This past Monday, Wesley had their Admissions Committee meeting after which I called and they said Mom was turned down for Upton Court, but accepted for Goodman Gardens. It turns out that Goodman does have a sort of 'in between' unit on the 6th and 7th floors. I went over to see it after work that day and it is very nice. They have all private rooms and you can bring in all your own furniture except the bed. The rooms were fairly big and the halls were large and bright and nicely decorated. There's a restaurant-looking dining room on the main floor or the residents can eat on their own floor. Each floor has its own dining room. The catch was that there are no vacancies and they have no idea when there will be one. Currently, there are two people in Upton Court waiting for rooms in Goodman Gardens, so that puts Mom third on the list. The wait could be weeks, maybe months. So I called the other place back on Tuesday morning and we made arrangements to bring Mom in for an interview that same afternoon.

Michelle was taking care of her that day and she brought her over to the nursing home and I met them there. Michelle told me later that she expected trouble because Mom had been agitated all day. Earlier in the day, Michelle locked the doors and went up to take a shower. She wasn't in the bathroom too long, but when she came out, she heard Mom making a commotion downstairs. She went down to find Mom had banged on the front window when the mailman went by, tried to get him to let her out and, by the time Michelle came down, the guy was at the back door trying to reassure Mom that he'd get her some help to get her out. Michelle was more than a little embarrassed.

We were both surprised to find that she was perfectly calm and happy when we all arrived to talk to the social worker. We talked in the woman's office first and then took Mom for a tour of the building. The social worker told Mom that the first part of the building was for people who needed a lot more care than she did, and where she was going to live, there were people like herself who were somewhat confused and had problems with their memories. From that point onward, she talked to Mom as if the move was an accomplished fact. Mom went along and smiled and agreed with everything.

June 13, 1991

We made the decision to go ahead with placement and stay on the waiting list at Wesley on East. That way, if things didn't work out well, we still had another option down the road. I had given it a whole lot of thought and decided that I was looking at the two facilities from my (semi) normal point of view and what appealed to me. I hadn't really considered what was best from Mom's point of view. Basically, I came to the conclusion that the program was more important than the aesthetics. This nursing home had a unit which focused on people with Alzheimer's. Once I decided, we moved fast. Michelle went out to the doctor's office Wednesday and got a report from there and hand-delivered it to the social worker. They called me that afternoon and said everything was in place. Mom would move in on Friday. Mom remembered meeting with the social worker and talked about it Tuesday evening and Wednesday, but not on Thursday. Friday morning, Sandy came over to help me move Mom's things, and Carolyn came to take Mom out. I told Mom it was Friday and this was the day she was going to move to her new place. She said, "What's that?" I told her Carolyn was going to take her out to breakfast and get her hair done and Sandy was going to help me with her things and we'd meet her there. Then to add a wrinkle to an already tense morning, Mom announced that she lost her purse, but for some reason, she didn't seem upset about it. It was weird because all she has to do is misplace a tissue and the house gets turned upside down till she finds it. This time, she didn't seem very concerned at all. Carolyn went in and looked in all her usual hiding places, but we didn't find it. So I just gave her some money and told Mom that Sandy and I would find it later. She went on her way without a complaint.

So Sandy and I got to work. I had borrowed a van from a friend of Gary's. Gary, by the way, was in NYC for the week at an IBM seminar and knew nothing of what was going on. Another friend, Mike, came over to help move Mom's dresser, chair and TV. We got everything packed, loaded and moved into her new room by about 10:30 a.m. and then Sandy and Mike left. At about 11:30 a.m., Carolyn showed up with Mom. The intake social worker was there to greet her and when we got inside, she introduced Mom to the unit social worker. I had met her earlier and went over some paperwork with her. She said she'd be back when Mom showed up to help get her settled in and take her around to introduce her to some of the other people on the unit.

I had asked previously how moving day would go and was told they like the resident and family to get there around 11:00 a.m. We would meet with the unit social worker, the nursing staff, the house physician, do some paperwork, and have lunch. Generally, the family leaves around 3:00 p.m. and then they take the new resident and help them get accustomed to the new environment.

What, in fact, happened was drastically different. We went up to the room. When Mom first saw all her things there, she acted as if she hadn't seen these things in a real long time. After a couple minutes of oohing and aahing, it all of a sudden hit her that if her things were in this place, then she must have to stay here. She was definitely not happy about that. Carolyn and I told her she'd have to stay and that she'd get used to it after a while. She objected off and on throughout the afternoon, but never really had a fit over it. At one point, she said to someone, "I want to go home, but THESE TWO (and she shook her fist at Carolyn and me) won't let me!" I'm pretty sure she thought she was in a hospital (it looked like one) and had no idea why.

I need to back track again. I keep remembering things that I meant to tell you along the way, but so much has happened in such a short time that I'm getting it all out of order. I mentioned earlier that the room was a double. I had been told that the other person they were interviewing for the room was a woman in the early stages of Alzheimer's. She lived alone and had no family and was admitting herself into the unit in anticipation of what was to come. By Friday, her lawyer had stepped into the picture and decided she was rushing into this decision and wanted her to look at other places, so if she came here, it wouldn't be for at least another week or so. Meanwhile, Mom had the whole room to herself. The two bright spots about this whole thing were the room, which was a corner room on the front of the building with two huge windows, and the lady across the hall who is just the sweetest thing. Her name is Isabelle and I stop to see her whenever I'm there if she doesn't come across herself to say hello. Aunt Nan has made friends with her too.

So anyway, the unit social worker stuck around for about ten minutes or so and then disappeared. Isabelle came over to introduce herself and shortly thereafter, the house doctor came to talk to Mom and do a cursory exam. After he left, a nurse came and stuck her head in to say a lunch tray would be up in about an hour, and that was about it. It was just after 12:00 by then. Carolyn and I waited and waited, expecting someone to come by, but no one ever did. About 1:00 p.m. Mom's lunch came up and while she ate, I went up to the nurse's desk and asked if the social worker was coming back. The nurse said no, that she was all through and I could go if I wanted to. I said I wasn't just going to leave Mom sitting down there all by herself. She was upset enough as it was. The nurse said not to worry about her; she'd be fine. There was some activity at 2:00 p.m. and if I thought Mom would like it, she could go. She wasn't sure what it was, perhaps a movie, but someone would be up between 1:45 and 2:15 to get everyone. I decided we would leave then. Well, 1:45 came and went and at 2:05, I went back to the desk and asked if the activities person would come to the end of the hall and get Mom. They assured me that they ask at every room if people are interested in going. At 2:20, no one had come yet so I headed for the nurse's desk once again. She said, "Oh, didn't anyone come for your mother?" So then they paged for someone to come and get her. When the woman came to get her, we said goodbye and she went off with a great deal of apprehension on her face. I went home less than thrilled, wondering whether they were going to stick her in this room at the end of the hall and forget about her.

The next morning, at about 8:30 a.m., I was awakened by the phone. It was the night nurse saying that Mom was very upset. She had gotten out of the building and was determined to walk home. The night before, they had put a Wanderguard bracelet on her ankle, but at about 8:00 a.m. when she got on the elevator and found her way to the front door, no alarm went off as she went outside. Fortunately, the guy at the front desk saw her go out and called the floor.

June 15, 1991

They had some trouble convincing her to come back in and when they did, they called me and put her on the phone. She was all bent out of shape and asking me to come right away and hurry; that I had to take her home. I kept telling her I would come to see her, but not right away; not till lunch time. Finally she gave the phone back to the nurse. In the background, I could hear someone saying, "No Bea. Don't do that. Bea, come over here. No, Bea." The nurse explained that she was trying to hang up the phone. The next thing I heard was a dial tone. A few minutes later, the nurse called back and as we talked, she sounded genuinely surprised at Mom's behavior – as if she had never seen anything like this before. She said, "Did she do this sort of thing at home?" Oh, and by the way, they found the ankle bracelet in her room. She had cut it off with a pair of scissors. This nurse went on to say that if she wouldn't wear the Wanderguard and kept getting 'combative' they would have to restrain her. At that point, I got bent out of shape myself and proceeded to tell her what I thought of their 'warm' welcome the day before and how really unimpressed I was so far. I was beginning to think they had one of two ways of dealing with residents – ignore them and hope they're quiet or tie them down if they aren't. She immediately apologized all over the place and said she was sorry that I had that impression and that they really do a good job and Mom would be well looked after and they would get her out of her room and they'd make every effort to see that she adjusted, etc.

Long about noon, Michelle and I went over and took lunch so we could take her outside on the back lawn to eat. When we got off the elevator, Mom was standing by the front desk talking to a gentleman resident and seemingly quite contented. She was thrilled to see us and more thrilled because we had found her purse. I told her we'd go out back to eat and she immediately invited the gentleman to join us. He said no thank you, that he was waiting for the streetcar to go home. (Michelle said one of these days I may come in and find her waiting for the streetcar with him).

We went out to eat in a pavilion they have in back and Mom happily went through her purse half a dozen times and ate her lunch. Every little while she'd ask if we could take her home, but didn't get upset when we said no. About an hour later, we went inside. When we got up to the floor, she said, "I'm not going back there." I said that Michelle hadn't seen her room yet, so she came along willingly in order to show it to her. We stayed for another half an hour or so and again, every now and then, Mom asked if we would take her home. At one point, Michelle said we couldn't because all her things were here. Then later Mom said, "You know what you should do? Go out to the desk and tell them we're going to take all this stuff out of here." – one of the truly longest string of intelligible words she had put together in quite a while. When I said I wouldn't do that, she tried to get Michelle to agree to take her home.

I need to back track here again. Last Wednesday evening, Michelle left for Pennsylvania where she's doing a summer research project at Lehigh University. That threw a wrench into the works because Mom was pretty sure at that point that she herself was moving somewhere. Now here was Michelle, packing her things and leaving too. When Michelle came back for the weekend, I suppose it made sense that she (Mom) could come back too. Michelle tried to tell Mom she couldn't take her home because she had moved to another place too where she had a room just like Mom's. Mom seemed to digest that, but we're not sure if it really made an impression.

Isabelle came from across the hall and visited a bit. I had seen her in the doorway of her room and waved, so she came scooting over saying, "I don't like to get in the way, but you DID wave." I assured her that she was welcome any time. Shortly thereafter, they came to take the residents to a bowling thing and Michelle and I made our exit. Mom went off a bit more readily than the day before.

During this visit, I talked to the day nurse, and told her that I did NOT want any restraints used on Mom and, if it was necessary, to give her a mild tranquilizer instead. When Aunt Therese first went to St. Ann's, they gave her tranquilizers for the first week or so. It took the edge off her anxiety while she got used to the environment and later, she didn't need them. The nurse said they had called the doctor that morning and that was what he recommended with my okay. She said they would not give them to her as a matter of course, but only on an as needed basis.

Sunday, I went up again right after lunch. The day nurse said Mom had had a bad evening and night, but not as bad as the night before. I had brought along a new zipper to replace a broken one on her purse. So I sat and did that while she puttered around in her room. She didn't ask me to take her home that day, but she seemed edgy and kept moving things around; pictures, clothes, odds and ends. The nurse had said that she had been trying to pack during the morning and I found a few clothes folded and stacked on her bed. Aunt Nan came in about an hour later and Mom barely acknowledged that she was there. After a bit, I suggested that we go out back and I'd leave and they could walk around the orchard. Aunt Nan had her dog, Yoda, in the car. It was a very warm day, so she went to get the dog while I took Mom outside. When they came back, I left. Aunt Nan told me later they were out for about an hour. She said their walk was slow because all the residents wanted to pet Yoda. After a while, Mom took the leash and walked the dog herself. Aunt Nan let them go a ways without her and when it looked like Mom was headed for someone's back yard, she called Yoda and they both came back. They went back in at Mom's request and went to her room where Mom got distracted and went into her puttering mode again. Aunt Nan took Yoda over to see Isabelle and then she and Mom walked down the hall to the TV room where everyone wanted to see the dog. Mom started talking to an aide and shortly later, turned to Aunt Nan and said, "I think you should take Yoda home." And that was that.

Monday, I didn't go up. Tuesday when I got home from work, Gary said that the nurse had called and said that Mom had had a bad day Monday. Gary asked if they wanted us to come up or do anything, but she said no, that she was just calling to let us know how things were going. Mom had had a $20 bill in her purse and was carrying it around, giving it to people and trying to get it back and generally upsetting the apple cart, so the nurse took the $20 away. I can pretty well guarantee that's why they had a difficult time with her Monday.

Anyway, I went up Tuesday evening. She was eating dinner when I got there. I said hi and she looked up at me as if I had been there all along. I sat with her while she ate and then suggested we go to her room because I had bought her stockings and wanted to put them away. It took some doing to get her away from her tray – trying to tidy up you know – but we finally headed down the hall. She had taken a little salt packet from the tray and wrapped it up in a napkin. She showed it to me and said, "I really like these things." Apparently so; I later found half a dozen or so hidden all around her room. They had a Mass at 7:30 p.m. in another part of the building so I took her to that. She was quite happy to go along and the priest was very good, obviously used to speaking to elderly people. When we came back, I asked her for any dirty clothes she might have so I could take them and launder them. I had to ask about 73 times before she got the idea and when she finally pulled out a few things, I said I had to go. She started objecting slightly and I said I would wash and iron her clothes and bring them back on Thursday. So she said okay and I left. She closed the door behind me and didn't follow me down the hallway.

Wednesday, the unit social worker called me at work and said they decided to move Mom into a private room. They had someone lined up to move into the double room with her but felt Mom needed more time to calm down. Then another person in a private room moved to skilled nursing so Mom moved to that room. Besides the fact that Mom had her fits of anger in the evenings, she was kind of spreading out in the double room, using the other dresser and putting her clothes on the other bed. They weren't too sure that she'd be willing to pull back and share. I figured the move would upset things all over again, but better now than later. Besides, a private room is what we wanted in the first place. They moved her Thursday. I went up after work to see how it went. I'm not sure if it was the move or the tranquilizers, but she was very subdued. She was moving things from here to there in the room, heavily into her puttering mode. I think it may have been beneficial in the fact that it gave her something to do.

When I got there, she was in the solarium with a whole group of other residents. One of the aides said they were concerned because her ankles were rather swollen. She and the nurse I talked to later said they felt it was because she was wearing shoes with a bit of a heel and that she walked all the time and rarely sat down. I assured them that this was normal. She ALWAYS wears shoes with heels and NEVER sits down. The nurse also said that Mom's B12 level and her hematocrit were low and they were going to give her B12 shots for a while to get it back up. I asked her if this could cause the swelling. She said it was possible, but if the swelling didn't go down after her blood count was up, they'd treat that separately. I tried to call the doctor the next day, but he never got back to me. What has me concerned is that she had a physical three weeks ago and her blood tests were normal. It doesn't seem right that she should have a problem this soon afterward. I'm going to call her outside doctor on Monday too. I talked to a nurse friend last night and she said it's possible that the tranquilizers could cause the ankle swelling and it should go away. Also, the swelling could cause the blood tests to appear low even when they're not because plasma moves to the site of the swelling. Wouldn't you think the nurses at the home would have come to the same conclusion?

One good thing came out of my visit Thursday night. When I talked to the head nurse for evenings, she said, "You know, I've been reading the chart on your mother every day and noticing all the comments about the difficulties she's had and the trouble, but I haven't had any problems with her at all. In fact, I think she's adjusting beautifully for only having been here one week. It's always a difficult time when someone comes in here new, but she's doing very well." It was really nice to hear someone from that place say something positive for a change. Except for that nurse, all the staff I've dealt with have been polite and I suppose they're trying to be helpful, but everyone of them has started off with a complaint when I talk to them. I keep getting the feeling that at any moment they are going to call and ask me to take Mom back. (Susan assured me this wouldn't happen, that this was not my child and I am not responsible for her behavior, but I still had my doubts).

June 18, 1991

New surprises (dilemmas?) every day! Yesterday morning I got a call from Wesley on East. Much to their surprise, and mine, they have a room available already at Goodman Gardens. It was a rare series of occurrences that cause three people to be moved all at the same time, but there it was. I don't exactly know what to do. I hadn't expected this call for weeks and I thought I'd have time to really assess the situation at the other place and decide whether or not to move Mom. I talked to all sorts of people in the last 24 hours, people at work, Susan, Michelle, Gary, David, a couple of people from St. Ann's, etc. and got all sorts of differing opinions. I'd change my mind with each one I heard.

When I talked to Michelle last night, I said I had the idea in my mind that Goodman Gardens was going to be this terrific place, different from any other. But maybe it wasn't. Maybe nursing homes were all alike and it would be no different from where she was now. Michelle said even if they were no different, it would make me happier and Mom would be no better or worse off than she is now. And too, having been through the process at the other place, I would know more what to look for and what questions to ask. Gary, on the other hand, thought we should leave her where she is. Of course, he hasn't seen either place, but I think he anticipates more anxiety for me – which would probably occur, but certainly not to the extent of the previous several weeks.

Finally, the last thing Monday night, I decided to go to a wiser head, so I called Aunt Nan to get her input and she had the best idea of all. Since we couldn't ask Mom what she wanted (she wouldn't understand the question, nor be able to formulate an answer), I should take her to Goodman Gardens and get a visual reaction and then decide. So that's what I did on my lunch hour today.

I went over to pick her up at noon. When I got there, Debbie was visiting. I told her I had to take Mom out right away and quickly explained why. I asked her if she had the time to come along and she readily agreed.

When we got there, Debbie and Mom stood in the lobby with their mouths hanging open as if they couldn't believe the place. It certainly is a far cry from a nursing home appearance. The intake social worker, and the unit social worker met us at the front door and took us up to the 6th floor. Once there, we met the nurse manager and a couple of staff members. The nurse manager is Irish – right from Ireland, accent and all. She struck me right away as the type who would definitely make me toe the line and would let Mom do anything she liked. I liked her immediately. The way she spoke indicated that she had a really good knowledge of and way with dementia patients. I told them all about Mom's problems at the other place so far and they kept reassuring me all of that is perfectly normal. I didn't want them to be shocked by her behavior. Not only were they not shocked, they weren't even concerned.

The 6th floor has about 23 residents and their policy is to maintain a very low-key, quiet environment. They've found that the residents respond much better and settle in to their new home more readily. The vacant room was a corner room fairly near the elevator (easy to locate for a confused person). We took Mom in to see it, and she reacted very positively. She looked all around, seemed delighted with the view from the window. They told her the bed was brand new and Mom sat on it and bounced a bit, getting the feel of it. The intake social worker said it was an electric bed and Mom jumped right off. She hurriedly assured her she only meant that it could move up and down. Then Debbie asked Mom if she'd like to live here rather than where she is now. She said, "Oh yes! But I could never afford a place like this!" We told her it was all paid for and she didn't have to worry about it. We think she thought it was a hotel of some sort, but whatever, she was very impressed. Before we left, we made arrangements to move her on Friday. I anticipate her welcome at Goodman Gardens will be considerably warmer than it was at the first place. I am VERY OPTIMISTIC!

June 19, 1991

As I had indicated before, the staff at the first nursing home had this rather unique way of making me feel guilty for something – I wasn't sure just what – but, with the exception of one evening nurse, they all complained. It was so odd, really, because this was a unit for people with dementia and the staff seemed to act as if they had no idea how to handle them, at least not a new, adjusting resident.

When I went back there on Tuesday to let them know about the move, I saw this look pass over the face of the day nurse, just for a split second that said she was pleased to be rid of Mom. If I hadn't been looking right at her, I wouldn't have seen it. The next day, when I called the intake social worker to find out if there was anything I needed to do before Friday, she asked me what had happened. I explained how this had come up so suddenly, much to everyone's surprise, how I had debated all Monday night and Tuesday morning, how I decided to take Mom to Goodman Gardens to get a visual reaction and how Mom really seemed to like it. I tried not to give the impression that we were pulling her out because of something they did, but rather that we were reverting to our first choice. Her response was, "Well, I have to be honest, we're all rather annoyed with you. Our entire staff did their best to make this work and your mother didn't make it any easier." I was so stunned, I didn't respond. She said I should talk to the unit social worker, not her and curtly said goodbye. Well, let me tell you, if I had ANY doubts about moving Mom at that point, they were totally gone after that remark. Sure, let's blame the 79-year-old woman with dementia when the staff doesn't know what they're doing. This woman also knew from day one that my first choice was Wesley and that we would be on the waiting list there. She assured me more than once that we could change our minds and move Mom at any time with three days notice.

Another note: the one nurse I met last week on evenings who didn't have any complaints about Mom – well, I saw her tonight and she said she heard Mom was moving. She said, "I can't say I won't miss your mother, but you're definitely making the right decision. I worked at Wesley for five years and it's excellent. It will be a much better place for your mother."

Debbie called me at work today to say again how pleased she is about the move. She said, "I'd put my mother in Wesley, and there's nothing wrong with her!" I also talked to Aunt Nan. She was so happy and relieved about the move. She said she didn't want to influence me either way, but she was thrilled that I chose to move Mom.

June 24, 1991

As another stroke of good luck would have it, Susan came up to help me move Mom. We moved her this past Friday, and I've been extremely pleased with the decision. It's like night and day between the two facilities. Susan and Gary were amazed at the contrast between the two the day we moved; from a noisy, crowded, hospital-like environment to a quiet, spacious, hotel-like environment. When we got there, we met with the social worker, Rachel, and she ended up spending about two hours with us. She was so sweet and helpful. Different staff members were in and out all while we were there, introducing themselves and saying hello to Mom. One girl brought a couple of other residents in to meet Mom. When we left, two staff members were taking Mom to lunch. Later that day, I called Rachel to see how things went after we left and she assured me not to worry, that Mom would be happy. And she abruptly said she had to go because she was going to escort Mom to a planned activity in about five minutes (not her job; just an extra kindness for a new resident).

June 25, 1991

Mom seemed to like the place right off the bat and within a couple of days accepted that this was now her home. By the same token, she didn't understand why she couldn't go out whenever she liked. I got a second hand report that she had taken off by herself one day, but came right back. I didn't get any subsequent reports or complaints about Mom's little stroll. I went up to see her after work tonight. She was grumbling about the terrible day she had had, but I couldn't figure out why. I got the impression they kept her busy with things because she kept saying ". . .all the things I had to do. . ." and ". . .what I've been through." She wasn't really upset, just sort of bugged. I noted on the calendar that Aunt Nan had been there earlier today and Carolyn and Debbie were there yesterday. Maybe that was a bit much for her, but overall, she was fine. I took her out for a short walk before dinner which she wasn't altogether thrilled about because there was a slight breeze and her hair got blown. As we were coming back, she saw the building ahead and said, "That's where I live."

June 29, 1991

A few days after Mom was there, I talked to one of the social workers and she said that whenever Mom got the urge to go walking, if anyone was free, they'd go with her. It turned out they'd just walk her around the block and she was more than satisfied to come back in. Nurses, aides, social workers, even the chaplain had gone out with her at various times.

One thing that has really impressed me about Wesley is that all the staff members seem to know all the residents; the security guards, the receptionists, the office people, they all get to know the residents. It's great. Now that she's been there a few days, Mom seems rather secure. Whenever they take her on an outing, or even when I take her out, within a fairly short time, she's anxious to get back. She has made friends with a woman across the hall from her. This woman is at about the same level of Alzheimer's as Mom and they seem to communicate with each other pretty well even though neither one makes sense to us. This woman was a clothing designer in her better days, so she and Mom have their sewing background in common. They visit back and forth and eat meals together.

Guess who called me a couple days ago? The intake social worker from the other nursing home! She had to talk to me to do an 'exit interview.' She asked how Mom was doing and then gingerly asked how I felt about her facility. She said they like to get an idea of how they can improve their services for others. First she asked what I liked about the place and then what I didn't like. I told her the one thing that drew me to it in the first place was that they had a unit specifically for people with dementia. Then I proceeded to tell her that in spite of that fact, the staff didn't really seem to know how to deal with them. I told her how, with the exception of one nurse, every other staff member greeted me day after day with complaints. While I knew they were trying to be helpful and keep me abreast of what was going on, I ended up feeling guilty that I had 'inflicted' her on them. I also told her about our infamous first day there and how little it resembled the picture she had painted for me. I forgot to mention the restraint thing. Anyway, I went into some detail and she seemed genuinely surprised, especially about moving in day. She said she really thought it was as she had described and there would be far more attention paid to new residents in the future. She said she appreciated my honesty and hoped things would work out well for us. She attempted to soften her comments of last week by saying that she was "discouraged" by our taking Mom out so soon when they "had worked so hard to get her in"(???), but hastened to add that I wasn't to take it personally. I think she got the message. Whether it makes a difference to the home as a whole, who knows.

June 30, 1991

Susan, I remembered what I wanted to tell you the other night. Our little floral victim that we tried to save from Mom's room never survived our less than genteel care. I let it sit on the kitchen windowsill with fresh water for a week and finally threw it away yesterday. It looked just as pitiful as when you were here only more dry. I suppose it's gone to that big arboretum in the sky. And, no, I didn't have a terribly ceremonious funeral for it. I dumped the stupid little green thing on it's dried little head and said, "Hah! That'll teach you to die on us you little weed!"

I got a letter (not a form letter either) from the chaplain at Wesley offering his services and help if we should so desire. Then I got a letter asking if I'd fill out a questionnaire about our impressions of the admission process. Gary got a phone call from the recreation department asking what kind of things Mom likes to do so they can offer some type of activity for her. (When he first heard it was someone from Goodman Gardens calling, he fully expected it to be a complaint of some sort about Mom. He was pleasantly surprised to find out it wasn't). He told them the only thing he could think of was sewing and the girl said that was great and they'd see how they could address that. I think I'll call tomorrow and see if they could make use of her portable sewing machine.

July 1, 1991

I took Mom shopping yesterday for shoes because she needs good walking shoes. What a mistake! Every store we went into, she headed right for the high-heeled, pointed toe dress shoes. Whenever I showed her comfortable shoes, she turned up her nose at them. Then, for some reason, when we were on our way out of the mall, in Sears, she spotted a display of nurse's shoes and made a beeline for them. I hastily encouraged her to try some on, but wouldn't you know, they didn't have her size. I ended up taking her back to Goodman and on my way home, stopped at another store and picked up a pair of nurse's shoes in her size. Tonight we were going out to dinner for our anniversary and Mrs. T's birthday, so I took the shoes along and had Mom try them on. They fit quite well and she likes them, so that task is done. However, I'm not at all sure she knows the shoes are hers. She kept trying to get me to try them on too.

July 21, 1991

Aunt June, just to fill you in, we just got back from a week in Colorado. Gary and I flew out and met Virginia & Bill, Carole & Jud, Tim & Kim, and Susan & Charlie. We had such a good time; relaxing, excellent weather, breath-taking scenery. I hated to see it come to an end. When we got back home, I stopped in to see Rachel and her first comment was that I looked much better than I had when she first met me.

Life seems to have gotten back to normal finally and I can actually enjoy it, knowing that Mom is in exceptionally good hands. I went up to see her today. Her initial reaction was as if I had been away for a while, but within minutes, she was acting as if I had been here all along. Carole, I decided to give her that book you gave me, "14,000 Things To Be Happy About." I thought it might be just the thing for her. She still can read words, but doesn't comprehend too much. Little one-liners might please her.

CHAPTER 11

Interlude between letters

Shortly after that last note, my letters became less frequent and reports about Mom of less urgency. Mom settled into Wesley on East so well, it's almost hard to remember a time when she wasn't there. I attended Family Council meetings as well as support group meetings that were held every other month.

As I reread these letters, other little vignettes come to mind, incidents that typify the behavioral changes and the 'unlearning' that was occurring.

When Mom was living with us, I took her to Church one day, and as we walked along the school hallway to the Church, we came upon one of the priests, Fr. Robert Hale, talking to a small child, maybe 5 years old, who was showing him a little book she had. Father was very kindly admiring it. Mom promptly pulled out her rosary and held it out and said, "See, I have this!" in the way another little child might have. Fr. Hale, without a moment's hesitation or even a passing look of surprise, turned and gently made an equal fuss over her rosary as he had over the book, and Mom went on her way happily. I can't express what that meant to me. The expectation was that people would be either startled or over-indulgent at Mom's child-like behavior. When those rare instances occurred that someone took her in stride and responded naturally, it touched my heart like nothing else could.

Michelle and David had one friend, Greg, who was exceptionally kind and easy going with Mom. Most of their friends were understandably rather uncomfortable and just didn't know how to cope with her. Greg was happy to be around her. It was always such a relief and help to me when people understood.

In her struggle to remember things, Mom wrote notes all the time. She frequently asked me for people's names and addresses so she could write them down. Once Mom moved into the nursing home, I found little notebooks all over the house where she had written down prayers, items she had bought along with their prices, people's names and who they were ("Patty's friend" or "David's friend" or "eye Doctor"). She had a list of things she wanted to bring when she moved to New York from New Mexico which included things like "picture of man with tears and beard," "picture of Pope – under first picture of Pope," and "winter coat in front closet off living room." There were notes that had meaning only for her such as "ready 5—50," "Jesus of Nazareth, Christ on page, Elizabeth."

Mom used to be a prolific letter writer, writing to me and others frequently from the time she and Dad first moved to New Mexico. During the last year before Mom moved back to New York, she stopped writing, mainly because we were in phone contact so often, but also because I think it was getting very difficult for her. Shortly after Mom had come to live with us, she attempted to write a letter to a friend in Florida to let her know she was now here in Rochester. I found these notes after Mom moved to Wesley.

"Dear Clara,

Our parts have spread far, far apart and I am so sorry for the breach.

Most of my family have dropped to "Myself" "Bea" and "June," out of seven children just us two.

We are back in Rochester, and I am living with June and she is still in her farm near Rush.

I am very happy with the David and Michelle people in the out of teen set and both of them are   "

(*My grandfather had a farm in West Bloomfield some 50 years ago*). She
started the letter over –

> "Our parts have spread far, far apart and I am so
> sorry for the breach. Most of my family had dropped to
> myself and June, out of seven just us two.
>
> We are back in Rochester, and I have went to live in
> with my youngest daughter and her brother – all are connected
> Manions.
>
> I am very happy and living in a beautiful house
> (small) built off of their home for me. I am writing this right
> now in it, I neglected to say a daughter and son, who both are
> in my home and their home also.
>
> I have many notes to write and want to get them out
> before too long.
>
> Bea"

Another time she attempted to answer a letter Virginia's daughter,
Radey, had written. I didn't realize she had sent it, and was rather surprised
she managed to address it correctly considering she signed it 'Radey.' I
would have expected her to address it to herself. Virginia sent me a copy
after having had a rather difficult time explaining it to Radey.

> "Dear Radey McKenna, Thompson
>
> I am so very delighted to have you and Radey and
> especially going into fifth grade in Rochester, New York.
>
> I do think the cow going across the road, and, be a
> grandaughter and because it was so funny for being the
> chicken's day off, and not being ready to grab it – the chicken
> was ready to grab it on the day off – so – he left it to
>
> grabbed it or some one did.
>
> "AND HAD – MIGHT FAST"
>
> "WE ALL WERE"

So we had a great laugh off of ours.

Well we had a home of time, so we did go to your home and had a red porch and black rocker, it was quite on the porches.

Then a purple hammock and chair. We went to their red house with a blue door and a snake all on the "outer" on the colors, beautiful blue, green, black snake.

Will will maybe again on wonders of the outdoor,

> Your grandaughter,
>
> Radey"

As I said, Virginia had quite a time explaining this to a 9-year-old.

In years Mom was at Wesley, there were many changes. For the first couple of years, I was able to take her out for ice cream or lunch or to shop around in stores. But by 1994, she wasn't able to sit still long enough to eat, and in the stores, she didn't realize that she couldn't take things off the shelves. So at that point, I would take her out just to walk or for rides in the car. In the nursing home, this constant need to walk created a problem at mealtimes. She wouldn't sit still long enough to eat. They tried giving her food she could carry around and that worked for a while, but in time, she quite forgot what was in her hand and either set it down someplace or would play with it. So they did their best to feed her 'on the run.'

During that time period, Mom was physically quite well. She no longer spoke with any sense. She just made repetitive sounds or spoke 'gibberish.' She only understood a little of what was said to her. She was constantly in motion as I've said, walking the halls day and night. There were curious contrasts in her behavior. On the one hand, she could be very distractible in that she wouldn't focus on any one thing for more than a few minutes. For instance, if you tried to show her pictures or tried to get her to watch TV or sit down and eat, within a few minutes she lost interest and was off and walking again. On the other hand, if she got focused on a paper napkin or doll or some other item she had in her hands, you couldn't distract her no matter how you tried. I once watched as she was tearing up a paper napkin into little pieces. A metal tray dropped to the floor behind her and, while I jumped a foot, she never even blinked.

Periodically, I would realize that because I viewed whatever her current status was as normal, or typical, other people had no idea what she was really like. Friends would say, "If you said such and such to her, what would she say?" or "What do you talk about when you visit?" It occurred to me that I had answered "How's your Mother?" with "Oh, she's fine," a little too convincingly. When she was still walking and I'd go to visit, we didn't sit down together and talk. I would go up mainly just to be there. I'd straighten up her room and her clothes, return any stray items she had taken from other rooms, and then I'd sit and read or watch TV. She'd be in and out of the room and I'd ask what she was up to or give her some candy. Sometimes she'd focus enough to realize I was there and would speak to me, but with no real words. Other times, she'd look right past me.

Even with my sisters, I was brought up short with the realization that I hadn't been keeping them up to date with the changes in her condition. One Christmas, they got together and had a gift sent to her, specially wrapped and decorated. When it arrived, I wasn't there. Later, the staff told me a package of foods and treats had come and they had put it in the refrigerator. I asked who it was from, but they didn't know. (I'm guessing there was a card which Mom promptly stowed away somewhere or lost). There were multiple small boxes of items, and I told the staff to be sure Mom got a portion of it and then to share it among the staff and other residents. Subsequently, I sent a note to my aunts and my sisters and told them about it. Well, as it turned out, when I realized how upset I had made my sisters by treating this gift so casually, I realized two things. First, I had treated the receipt of the gift very badly, and second, I had fallen way short of keeping them informed. At that point in time, Mom had little awareness of her surroundings. You could get right in front of her and call her name or say, "Here, look at this," and you might as well have been invisible. She'd look right past you. Hence, the lovely packaging would have been lost on her. And while she would (and did) enjoy the treats, if the staff left them in her room, they would have been carried all over the place and left heaven knows where.

Awareness of her environment came and went. Often she'd look up and smile when I came in the room. From time to time she'd 'talk' to me with inflections in her voice that suggested she really had something to say. I just responded to the tone of her voice and she seemed satisfied. But there were still times when she'd look right through me as if I weren't even in her field of vision.

I gave her a baby doll dressed in a fur snowsuit and it almost looked real. I thought she'd take to it instantly. I also brought along a plastic rose that day. She totally ignored the doll, took the rose and tore it into pieces, pulling all the leaves off and then the petals. It kept her busy for some time. Sometimes I have no clue. As it turns out, however, after I left, she made acquaintance with the doll and it's been her constant companion ever since. Everyone knew that was Bea's baby and it went wherever she went.

In the spring of 1994, Mom started experiencing these occasional jerking motions. You know how it feels when you're just drifting off to sleep and you dream that you're falling and your whole body jerks? Well, that's what it was like. They're called myclonal jerks. At first they were pretty infrequent, but it occurred with more regularity as time went on. If she was standing when it happened, she was apt to fall. The doctor suggested it could be the tranquilizer she was on. They decided to gradually reduce it, and if she did all right without it, they'd keep her off. But for some reason, before they even got to ground zero with the one drug, they started her on another one and never stopped to see if she needed it. However, the jerking stopped so I left well enough alone. About 4 or 5 months later, it started again. I immediately asked the doctor to stop her other tranquilizer. She was reluctant because she felt it was the disease, not the drug, but she agreed to try. With the end of that drug, the jerking motions stopped again, but this time only for 2 or 3 months. When they started again, we started to see a pattern. They would start most often in the morning, they'd occur every few minutes for an hour or so, and then stop. Mom would usually sleep for a while after each spell. So the staff would watch her closely each morning. If they saw any sign of a problem, they'd put her in a geriatric chair and keep her there till it stopped. Then they'd let her go and she'd be fine the rest of the day.

That was a good solution for a while, but we knew it was only a matter of time before the frequency would increase. We had no idea how we were going to keep her down all the time. She had fallen several times – once a fall sent her to the hospital for stitches. Once, she didn't quite fall, but dropped her baby, and she wept so sadly over that. It was heartbreaking. Another time, one of the nurses was walking toward Mom when she jerked and fell, breaking open her stitches. The nurse felt just awful that she couldn't reach her in time to catch her. It was a terribly stressful time for all of us.

But God steps in when we have no answers. Around February of 1995, Mom 'forgot' how to walk. It happened all of a sudden. You'd sit her down in a chair, and while she might work her way forward to the edge of it, she wouldn't get up. The connection from her brain to the muscles in her legs just wasn't there any more. If we helped her up, she could walk with assistance, but she couldn't get going on her own. And the blessing on top of that was she didn't seem to mind. From that day on, she was remarkably more content than I had seen her in years.

She eventually reached the point where she didn't walk or talk, and she couldn't do things for herself. In fact, on days she was tired or not too alert, she couldn't even move herself from whatever position she was in. I went to Wesley frequently to feed her lunch or dinner. She had an amazing appetite – especially for sweets.

I told a friend once that I had reached the point where I couldn't remember what Mom was like before Alzheimer's. She said that I would remember after Mom was gone. Then the years of her illness would fade into the background and all of her good years would be clear again. It has occurred to me that this may actually be beneficial. Time and again, people would say to me that it must be so hard to see my Mother like this, but since that was the only reality, it wasn't that hard. Going to the nursing home was just part of my normal routine and Mom's condition was 'normal' too. In fact, the only way I had of measuring how she was changing was to think where we were perhaps six months previously.

Did I feel guilty about placing Mom in a nursing home? You bet I did. Back in April of 1991, when I had "come to the end of my rope," and actually gave my first serious thought to nursing home care, I felt so guilty that I went to a psychologist to help deal with the stress and guilt. The day I moved her in, I found myself walking an emotional tightrope. On the one hand, I was excited at the prospect of knowing that before the day was over, I would have my freedom back and the tranquility of being able to eat and sleep and come and go without worry. On the other hand, I felt guilty about being glad, and terribly downcast that circumstances had brought us to this point. There are times when I can't help but think I should have been able to cope better, to give her the physical and emotional care she needed and deserved. But then I have to bring back to mind those last weeks before placement and remember how difficult it was for her as well as for myself. The guilt is less acute and less frequent as time goes on, but every now and then it crops up unexpectedly.

Somewhere along the way, I read an interesting perspective on nursing home placement for people with dementia. For the dementia patient, one of the few things that helps them cope and remain on an even keel is consistency. In your average family household, this can be very difficult to maintain with people coming and going at different times, company dropping in, the phone ringing, etc. In a nursing home setting, it's very reassuring for someone who's struggling with memory to be in an unchanging environment. Meal times, bedtime, activities are, for the most part, the same every day. There are fewer disruptions for a confused mind to have to process. From that perspective, there comes a time when it's actually better for an Alzheimer's patient to be in a structured environment rather than at home.

Over the years, Alzheimer's became a fact of life for me. I lived with Mom's disease for over twelve years. Also, spending so much time with other folks at the nursing home with dementia, it became pretty routine after a while.

CHAPTER 12

The letters resume as the end approaches

January 17, 2000

We had an issue with Mom recently. It took us over a week to put together what happened, but it finally got resolved. A week ago, one of Mom's regular caregivers, Dora, wheeled her back to her room after dinner. Some time later (maybe an hour), Dora went to put her to bed. When she took the tray off the chair, Mom immediately slid out and it was all Dora could do to catch her and haul her up into the bed – 100+ pounds of dead weight. But she did, and Mom was fine; we thought. Friday night, I was there for dinner and Dora told me about the incident, but didn't say what night it happened. Saturday, I got a call from the nurse saying they had found a couple bruises on Mom's chest. She was fine, but they wanted me to know. Sunday I went in and the aide showed me the bruises. Startling is an understatement. She had a bruise all the way across her chest, in every shade of red, purple, black and blue. All of us had the same reaction, that it was the tray from her chair. She leans forward a lot, but we couldn't figure why it didn't get reported before Saturday. It was huge. On Monday, we talked to Tammy and she said there was nothing there Friday morning. Then we talked to Michael who had her Thursday, and he insisted there was nothing on his shift. I mentioned to them what Dora had told me and Michael said that must have happened on Tuesday because that was when Dora was working. But that didn't make sense. There's no way a bruise like this wouldn't have been visible for four days. On the other hand, I have complete trust in these people and they wouldn't lie. We were left with just writing it off to the tray on her chair, and of course, they got her a new chair without a tray. Finally, I saw Dora again this past Friday. She was beside herself over the incident. She said, "You know that no one here would ever hurt your Mother!" I assured her that I trusted them completely, but said that I just couldn't understand the time frame. Well, it turns out, Mom slid out of the chair on Thursday, not Tuesday. Apparently, for a time, her whole weight was pressing against the tray, and when Dora came for her and removed the tray, she went down. The bruises didn't show up till Friday night. Dora said when she saw them Saturday, she got hysterical and called for a nurse. She was frantic till she found out that it had already been reported. She was so afraid that she had caused this, but the nurse said no. She would have had to grab Mom from behind to cause this type of bruising. Tammy told me a couple days later that they were all upset, but Dora was the most upset. She was in tears over it. Tuesday, I called Mom's doctor and the nurse there said the nursing home had also just called. A staff doctor took a look and said the bruising appeared to be healing fine. There was no sign of pain when the aides moved Mom around, so there was practically no chance of a broken rib.

Not a pleasant incident, but I'll tell you what – it truly confirmed my confidence in her caregivers. I even had a couple of aides on the floor who don't take care of her express their concern. They're good people.

February 7, 2000

Mom has had a cold the past week or two and yesterday, a nurse from Wesley has called to say she was running a pretty high fever (>101). They suspect a urinary track infection and were going to start her on an antibiotic and do a urinalysis Monday (today). I went up today and she was doing better. Her temp was down to 99 and she was pretty alert. Tammy said she ate pretty well this morning too. She had been slowing down in that department for the past several days.

Looks like she's going to bounce back from this pretty well, but it got me thinking again that it can't be much longer before something comes along that will get the better of her.

February 13, 2000

Mom is sleeping more and more, and her appetite is decreasing somewhat. So what I'm thinking is that we should probably get more specific about what we want to do regarding funeral arrangements when she dies. As I'm sure I've told you, I set up a pre-paid funeral account when she went on Medicaid. That covers a good chunk of the costs – casket, outer liner, marker, cemetery plot and internment ($2775). Then she had a burial account at Citibank. They allow $1500 in an interest bearing account, and it's now $1834. Now, assuming the funeral home doesn't try to pull a fast one, like saying, "Gee, we don't have that casket any more. You'll have to pay a bazillion dollars for this one over here," we should be pretty close to covering what we need. I'm figuring on a burial rather than cremation because she was always rather put off by the very idea of cremation. Is there anything you'd like to have done? Let me know if you have any ideas or thoughts about this, okay?

I think I've also told you that some time back, maybe 6 or 7 years ago, I enrolled Mom in a research study with the University of Rochester. It entailed someone coming to 'interview' her once a year, and they got input from me on her progress. At the time of her death, they are going to do an autopsy. I mainly signed her up because I really wanted an autopsy to determine whether this is Alzheimer's or possibly Lewy Body Disease (which is less common and possibly not inherited). Hospitals charge an arm and a couple of legs to do an autopsy. With this, the cost is covered by the research group. When Mom dies, the funeral director will take her to UR and they will do their thing and transport her back to the funeral home.

Then, what I was thinking was that we wouldn't have any calling hours, but just a funeral Mass and a lunch or whatever here afterwards. But that's just my thought and certainly open to your thoughts or ideas. So what do you think? I'm anxious for any input you guys may have because I don't want to think about details at the eleventh hour. Oh! And by the way, I found Mom's will. I had said to Gary that I knew exactly what was in it, but he said he seriously doubted whether that would stand up in probate court. They generally don't accept "But I know exactly what was in it!" as legal and binding. Anyway, it says that her entire estate (and we use the term VERY loosely here) is to be divided among the four of us and if any of us dies before she does, our share goes to our children. Carole and I had kind of figured we'd each end up with about $2.59. When I told Michelle, she said, "David and I will fight over that extra penny, you know." I said if I was dead I wouldn't care. And Susan, you are listed as "Personal Representative" of the estate, and if you should choose to decline acceptance of this honor, Bill is your back-up or understudy or whatever.

February 19, 2000

Mom's now got a yeast infection which was caused by the antibiotic which she took for the UTI which was caused by the cold which caused the cold sores on her mouth, all of which contributed to the bedsore – "which lived in the house that Jack built."

March 23, 2000

After I sent you my last e-mail about Mom, I got to thinking that maybe it wouldn't be a half bad idea to have calling hours before the funeral. David pointed out that some people prefer to come to a funeral home rather than to Church, or as well as Church, so they can actually greet you. Oftentimes, the Mass is scheduled such that working people can't go anyway. As coincidence would have it, about the time I had written last, I had a Hospice patient whose family I had gotten to know pretty well. They were terrific people and when the gentleman died, I looked for the notice in the paper. I found they were just having a funeral Mass on a weekday, no calling hours. So the best I could do was send them a Mass card and note. I really was disappointed that I couldn't see them one more time to express my sympathy in person. Just another thought. What do you think?

March 29, 2000

Okay, so here's the scoop. I had kind of anticipated that Mom wouldn't make it through this whole year -- I doubted she'd see another birthday anyway. But it may be sooner than I thought. It's really hard to tell just now. In mid-January (I think I've told you some of this), she got a cold that hung on for about two weeks -- very unusual for her. She typically doesn't get sick or if she does, throws anything off within a day or two. This one really got her down. As a result, she also got a urinary infection. She was put on an antibiotic, Sipro, which, in turn, caused a yeast infection, which, in her case, caused her to get a rash from head to toe. The treatment for that acted quickly, thank goodness, and it all eventually cleared up.

However, also in January, they got her a new chair because the previous one had a tray on it and because she leans forward, she was getting bruised from the tray. So they got her a reclining geriatric chair and filled it with nice soft cushions and pillows. Well, because she had to have it reclined so she wouldn't pitch forward and because she can't move around herself, she managed to get a bedsore right at the base of her spine. (I saw it. It was horrid). Mind you, she has been off her feet for about 6 or more years and never had any skin problems at all. Well, two of her best caregivers, Tammy and Dora, set about getting rid of this thing. Meanwhile, I went to a surgical supply place and talked to a guy who really knew his stuff. The first thing he told me was not to be too shocked at its appearance because these things start on the inside and work their way out so that by the time it's noticed, it's already quite deep. Then he said to get rid of all the stuffing in her chair. He said it would seem as though this would be a good thing, but it was the worst thing for her. It made her even more immobile. She needs a firm surface. He sold me a square cushion for the seat of her chair with a 'V' cut-out in the back so that when she sat, her 'tailbone' wouldn't touch the chair. So I took the cushion in and the staff thought it was great. Tammy and Dora kept her in bed most of the time, though, and turned her every hour on the hour, kept her off her butt and made sure she was moved around enough not to risk pneumonia. Well, within two weeks, the thing was just about healed. I didn't think a bedsore could heal that quickly.

However -- once she was doing better, the staff started putting her in the chair more frequently. They used the cushion all right, but they put the soft padding up the back of the chair and they covered everything with layers of sheets which basically counteracted the cut-out in the seat cushion. Needless to say, the thing opened up again. Tammy and Dora were awfully upset (they didn't put her in the chair -- it was other aides who did). I called the nurse manager and told her the chair was evil and I didn't want her in it any more. She promised to get someone from physical therapy up to evaluate her for the best alternative. I highly doubted that because three or four staff people had said that back in January and it never happened. She also said they'd only put her in the chair when it was needed, like at meal times. I asked why meal times because I had been feeding her in bed. She said, "Well, that's fine when you're here, but when you're not, the girls have to have her in the dining room." Subsequently, I talked to four of the aides and they all said they feed her in bed and are happy to do it.

Now, to add to the mess, Mom's doctor called me a week ago and was fit to be tied. She had been in for a routine check-up and discovered the bedsore which she had never been called about and not only that, but the doctor at the home had been seeing her about this thing and "decided" that they should let the bedsore have its way and put her on Hospice. Well, I told Dr. Tarkington that, first of all, I was shocked that she hadn't been called, second that I didn't want the staff doctor anywhere near Mom and I would see to that, and thirdly, that even though I know she'll be ready for Hospice in the not too distant future, I didn't feel it was appropriate for her just now. Dr. T. was relieved to discover we were on the same wavelength and said she had cultured the sore and put Mom on an antibiotic.

The next day, I went in prepared to rant and rave at the nurse manager only to find that Dr. T. had done a pretty good job of that already. She was all apologies and assurances that Mom's case would be watched far more closely and she would be in touch weekly with the doctor and myself. I told her I didn't want the staff doctor to be making ANY decisions for Mom, and unless protocol absolutely demanded it, he wasn't to see her at all. She agreed.

But that's not all. Guess what antibiotic Mom got again, because no one had charted the fact that Mom is sensitive to Sipro, so Dr. Tarkington didn't know it. You guessed it! And guess what she got -- yup; another yeast infection and overall body rash. Once again, they treated for that and it has cleared up.

Today, the Nurse Manager caught up with me and said that Mom hadn't been eating or drinking at all well for a few days. I said she ate fine when I fed her Sunday. Monday, I wasn't there at meal time, but she seemed fine. She said some of the aides have been having trouble getting her to eat and drink so maybe we should put her on Hospice after all. I asked what the chances are that the antibiotic is upsetting her stomach. Also, she doesn't eat if she's not fully awake. Also, she doesn't eat well if they try to clean her mouth out first (they use a medicated rinse to keep her from getting gum infections -- she hates it). Also, there are some foods she doesn't like and will spit out and she's not at all keen on most vegetables any more. She said they would wait a little while to see if she comes out of this 'slump' and then we'd talk. She left. I set about feeding Mom dinner and she happily ate creamed chipped beef, green beans, chocolate cake, ice cream, cranberry juice and Boost (a nutritional drink).

The bottom line is that all these little things are adding up to break down her resistance and if much more accumulates, Hospice will be in order. However, I'm still not ready to say 'uncle' just yet. She's still eating, hasn't lost weight, and there hasn't been anything huge knocking her down. It seems these are mostly comfort issues, and I want them to treat them as best they can so she isn't in pain, or itching, or sore or whatever. I've been with Hospice for 14 years. I just don't think she's eligible quite yet. Hopefully, I'm not too biased here to make a good decision. If Dr. T. says to go for it, I will. Or if I say it's time, she'll go along with me. But no one else will make that decision. I'll keep you posted.

It seems more has happened with Mom in the last 3 months than in the last 8 1/2 years doesn't it?

April 01, 2000

Susan, thanks for your voice message today! It really brightened my day. In fact, when I heard it around noon, I left it on there, and when I came home a second time around seven, I played it again. Made me smile. I appreciate the 'kudos' (funny word -- I wonder where it comes from), and I know you guys would have done as much if Mom had chosen Arizona instead of New York back when.

Your delightful message has triggered some thoughts so I figured I'd send them along. I spoke a bit about this to Carole when I was out in Dec. It may sound a bit odd on the surface (especially if I don't explain it well), but it's really not. Mom's having been here over all these years has been God's greatest gift to me. There have been so many good things that have come from it and they're not all tangible or explainable. I have grown and changed in certain ways that I never would have believed possible. My 'scientific' self has watched this disease with fascination as she regressed through the various developmental ages. My 'daughter' self has become more caring and competent especially due to the encouragement (perhaps more accurately, the shoving and nagging) of the nursing home staff. If you had asked me eleven years ago, or nine or seven or even five, if I would EVER do any physical care for Mom, I would have said there was no way on this earth; not my thing; never going to happen. Now I do all sorts of things for her (some not so pleasant, I might add) and don't think anything of it. If you recall, by the time I placed her in the nursing home, I was about ready to kill her or at least, damage her severely. Well, the staff there freed me from that kind of stress and allowed me to learn to like her again and love her again. They took on all the things I couldn't do. Then, as time went on, different ones encouraged me to try simple things -- come during meals and just sit with her while she ate; give her a drink now and then; feed her ice cream -- little by little getting me more and more involved in her care. At the same time, I was getting to know and spend time around all the other residents. Well, I was a VERY, VERY slow learner. I see some people come in and lift and move their family member around and do all sorts of things for them right off the bat and I marvel at their capacity for caring. Nevertheless, because I had the good fortune to have an extended span of time, I was able to reach a level of giving her comfort care that I never would have dreamed I could do. Of course, lifting her isn't on the list because trying to move 100lb of uncooperative weight isn't easy. I can help the aides do it though.

I had a hospice patient about a year ago who had some dementia and had a stroke. While in the nursing home, he had a 2nd stroke. He stopped eating and drinking. The wife said, "They (nursing home and hospice staff) want to just let him go. They say that it's better this way. But I think if we could only get liquids into him, he'd feel better. Maybe he'll die anyway, but I think he'd be more comfortable." I told her she had to make the decision because they didn't have the emotional attachment that she did. As long as he was alive, in whatever state, he was still hers. She held him in her heart and had to make the decisions she could live with. She told the staff she wanted him on IV fluids, so they reluctantly moved him to a hospital. I went to see them there the next day, and he was resting comfortably, no longer with dry, raspy breathing. She was contented and ready to accept it if he died. He didn't. He not only perked back up, but he went home -- to their home. He's still alive today. (Turns out he was depressed about being in the nursing home).

The reason I tell you this is not because of what happened to him, but I realized that I was talking about myself as well. Mom is 'mine.' She's always glad to see me, and I'm always glad to see her. What more could you ask for? People have expressed all sorts of sympathy to me over the years, and I know their thoughts are kind, but I always come away with a kind of wonder at what they're sorry about. Mom has been, for the most part, physically well, and for the last six or more years, she has been generally very happy. She's not what most people consider 'fine' but that's what I always say when they ask. She is what she is. Life is what it is. You can't waste time wishing for what isn't. So, you just adapt and are happy. I sing to her, read to her, make faces at her which she imitates. If there's a down side to it, it's that I haven't really made it clear to others how she really is. When I realize that, I try to explain what I mean as 'fine' and say that she is WAY advanced down the road of Alzheimer's. But no one else ever sees her. Gary never goes up, nor does David nor do they ever ask about her. Michelle goes with me when she can, but that amounts to about once a year maybe. When the topic of Hospice came up these past couple of weeks, Gary and some of our friends were shocked which, in turn, suprised me. I mean, she's reached the level of about a 3 month old. How much farther can she go? The expectation, I guess, is that I should be in a state of mourning over this. But while the grief or mourning that goes along with the losses of Alzheimer's is the same as that experienced with death, divorce, losing a job, etc. etc., you can't -- physically or mentally -- hold on to grief for years. It's just not possible.

Mom has made me a much better volunteer for Hospice and the Alzheimer's Association because I know much of what the families and the patient are going through. Because I have learned and read so much about Alzheimer's and spent so much time with her 'nursing home family,' I've had the opportunity to really get to where these people are and, in turn, to try to explain that in presentations to hospice volunteers, family members at the nursing home, chaplains and women's groups. And as a pure bonus, Mom has gotten my foot in the door with many hospice families. When I go to see a new patient, sometimes the family responds with resistance or disinterest because of sheer exhaustion. When I say my Mother is also in a nursing home and has been for 9 years, all of a sudden, they let their guard down and 'let me in' because we're on the same wavelength. I'm not just another outsider trying to 'help.' I'm in the same boat trying to help.

I've made some absolutely terrific friends at the nursing home, mostly the aides. They are like family. One of her primary caregivers was actually in tears over Mom's recent problems. One thing I'm sorry about since Mom's been in bed all the time is that I don't get to sit in the dining room visiting with everyone any more. I've also discovered over the years that when there's a problem, you don't go to the administration, the supervisors, even the nurses. The aides have the answer every time. They're Mom's first line of defense, and if they care about the residents, they'll do anything for them. And they really do care.

I guess I've rambled on long enough. It's hard to put the whole big picture into words. What it boils down to is that God does what He does, or allows what He allows all for a good reason. We might not see that reason at first, or sometimes ever, but we have to trust. I read a book about Fr. Walter

Cizek, a Polish priest who spent the better part of his life during and after World War II in Soviet prison camps experiencing unimaginable suffering. He said he spent much of his life before and while he was in Siberia trying to figure out why he was there, unable to carry out his priestly duties (although he did a lot in secret). Didn't God call him to the priesthood, after all? He tried for a long time to figure out what God's will for him was before discovering that "the circumstances in which I found myself were God's will for me." That, to me, is one of the most profound statements I've ever read. It's not what you do, it's how you live the life into which you have been placed.

Oh! and by the way, Mom ate dinner just fine the past four nights. I think she just wasn't feeling well the previous few days due to the infection and the antibiotic and all. She's been very awake and alert these nights. Now, tonite, she didn't eat as much as usual, but she did eat some of everything and drank quite a bit.

May 6 2000

Mom seems to have reached another plateau of sorts (and has made the promoters of hospice eat their words). She doesn't eat nearly as much as she used to, but she eats enough considering that she doesn't move around. They were concerned that she wasn't drinking enough but the problem was she was getting really tired of cranberry juice. When I had her switched to thickened juices, all they ever gave her was apple juice for lunch and cranberry for dinner. She used to like cranberry – every now and then. Imagine having it every day! So I finally went out and bought a whole bunch of fruit nectars; apricot, pear, peach, etc. The international food section at Wegmans has 7 or 8 different kinds. The nectars are thick enough for her to manage pretty well. Then I found some mixed berry "Juicy Smoothies" in the baby food section. So I brought all this stuff in and told the girls to give her these and ignore the cranberry. She's been drinking fine ever since.

June 20, 2000

Thought you'd like to hear the latest from the wonderful world of the nursing home. I got a call about a week and a half ago from the nurse manager saying that the dentist had been in to see Mom for her annual check up. He reported that she has some fractured teeth and he recommended that all her teeth be pulled. He could sedate her and do it right there at Wesley. Well, I wasn't too kicked about the idea. I tried for a couple of days to reach the nurse to no avail. Meanwhile, I talked to an evening nurse and asked to see the report. The dentist wrote, "Excessive decay and fractured teeth. Patient uncooperative." How stupid is that!? He could have written, 'Patient UNABLE to cooperate.' Bit of a difference. The nurse didn't know anything about the dentist, nor did he sign the report, but she looked up in the general records and gave me his name. Monday I looked him up in the phone book, but he wasn't listed. One of the aides said he had seen him from time to time and he looks really old. Maybe he's retired and just does this on the side.

Turns out this dentist recently recommended pulling out all the teeth of another resident on Mom's floor. Her family agreed and after it was over, her mouth – of course – was all swollen and sore and she couldn't eat. Even after the soreness went away, they couldn't get her to eat because eating without teeth requires a whole different 'set of mechanics' and she couldn't figure out how to do it. Demented people can't learn stuff. This other lady is now on Hospice.

I called my dentist and he kind of hedged all around trying to avoid criticizing another dentist whom he didn't know, but the long and short of it was, he wouldn't do it. In fact, I had asked his opinion about Mom a long time ago. He said for someone in her condition, you'd be hard pressed to find a dentist who would be willing to pull all her teeth because it would be surgery under anesthetic and there's a good chance she couldn't tolerate it.

So I called Dr. Tarkington, who apparently then call the dentist in question, who called me. He said, "I've examined your Mother and found she has quite a bit of decay and I think it would be advisable to extract all her teeth. Since she has a behavioral problem – (moron!) – we'd have to sedate her to do the procedure or else we'll have to take her to Strong and put her under general anesthesia. Which way do you want to go?"

I said, "Now wait a minute. Let me ask you first if this is necessary at all." He said, "Well, if you don't want to have it done, we don't have to." As you can see, he was a hard sell. He went on to say that since she doesn't seem to be having any pain or discomfort, and since she eats well, there wasn't a real need to do this and I could get in touch with him some other time if I decide it becomes necessary. Something tells me that if it comes to that, I'll bring in another dentist.

I called Dr. T's office back. The nurse said when she informed Dr. T the day before of what I had said, her response was, "She's not seriously considering doing this is she?" They were very glad I decided against it.

Other than that, everything is on a nicely even keel with Mom. She is eating very well again, although she would be much happier if I would give her primarily ice cream and skip the vegetables altogether. (Sometimes I do!)

August 26, 2000

Mom's holding her own, quite stable, eating fairly well. Ever since she got over all her January thru March problems, she's been on a pretty consistent plateau. Looks like she may see 89 after all. She surprises me.

CHAPTER 13

The dying process begins

January 8, 2001

Looks like I'm going to have to rethink Mom's funeral Mass (whenever that may be) again. Fr. Zimmer died yesterday. Gary and I had asked him some months ago if he'd do the Mass when the time came.

Mom's roommate is on Hospice now. Real nice lady. If Mom outlives this one, that'll be six she's gone through.

January 18, 2001

They told me a couple days ago that Mom's lost about 10 pounds recently. (You couldn't prove it by me. She still feels like she weighs a ton when I try to move her!) She still eats well. Could be her digestive system is slowing down and the food's just not being processed. I'll let you know if there are any other changes. No other problems right now.

February 16, 2001

It's almost over. Then again, I thought that was the case last winter too. In March, around Mom's birthday, I had written to say that Mom would probably not see 89. She had so many problems at the time, but surprise! She got past them all and stabilized again. But once again, the social worker has suggested I put Mom on Hospice. She recently lost about 10lbs. but is still eating well. Her digestive system may be shutting down. I asked what else and was told there's nothing else, but how much further can she deteriorate. Certainly a good point.

After talking to her doctor and a friend who is a Hospice nurse, I decided against it. At this point in time, there's not a lot they can do for her and why stretch their resources unnecessarily. The only benefit would be the extra attention she'd get by having aide service every day and another nurse overseeing her care. She's not in any pain, nor does she have any concurrent illnesses. Besides which, when I brought up the idea to Mike, Dora and Tammy, they all said they didn't like the idea. I think they would see it as my lack of faith in their care. And it occurred to me (I've seen it happen) that once a person goes on Hospice in a nursing home, the whole tenor of their care changes. There's a sort of depression that settles on the environment and a sense of, "Oh well, nothing more to be done for her." There can also be a bit of tension between the Hospice staff and the nursing home staff; the Hospice staff thinking, 'We know Hospice patients better than they do,' and the nursing home staff thinking, 'We know this resident better than they do.' I don't want that for her right now. Her aides are more than capable of keeping her comfortable and treating whatever needs treating.

A couple of weeks ago, when I was wiping her mouth after dinner, I thought I heard a snapping sound. I checked to see if there was a broken tooth, but couldn't find anything. Since then, she has had a sensitivity on that side of her mouth and she hasn't been eating too well. Concurrently, I found out, she was put on an antibiotic for a yeast infection. It has dried up the mucous in her mouth. She doesn't drool as much as she did, but her mouth and lips are getting dried out. So with that combination of things, the poor eating isn't surprising. The last couple of days, she has eaten a little better, but not nearly as much as she used to.

Yesterday, while I was feeding her, she didn't open her right eye for quite a while. When she finally did, she had it open for a few seconds, then squeezed it shut and started to have a series of tics on that side of her face for several seconds. All I could think of is that it was like a mini-seizure. It finally stopped, and she opened her eye, but then fell asleep shortly thereafter.

She is less and less able to move on her own. If they lay her out in bed, in short order, she curls up. When I put her doll on the bed where she can see it, she smiles and tries to talk to it. She also moves around a bit as if touch it, but she can't move her arms or hands very far, nor can she grasp something even if it is within her reach.

She still smiles and responds visibly to my presence. Occasionally, she looks across the room smiles at something I don't see.

March 5, 2001

I got to Wesley and back without being eaten by a snowdrift. Actually the worst of this storm isn't supposed to hit till after midnight, but there were a few people slipping and sliding out there this afternoon.

Mom was pretty much out of it when I got there. When I started to clean her mouth and put some Chapstick on her, she felt really warm so I took her temp. It was 101.8. I told the nurse who said she'd give her some Tylenol. When she realized she couldn't give it to her by mouth, she said she'd have to have a nurse manager okay giving her a suppository. The nurse manager came from some other floor and said she'd have to call the doctor to see what she wanted to do. She asked if I wanted her moved to the hospital and I said no, unless Dr. Tarkington had a really good reason to do so. When I explained Mom's recent history, she agreed.

As it turned out, we got an on-call doctor who said to give the suppository, take a urine sample to check for infection, push fluids and call the next day. So she finally got the Tylenol, but we can't exactly push fluids on someone who won't wake up.

The hospital would probably test for infection and put her on IV fluids, but I'm not sure it would help at this point. My instinct is that this is just part of the dying process. If she had been eating well all along and was normally wakeful and got this fever, I'd say it was worth aggressively treating. I don't want Mom moved to a hospital just to have her die there. If she's going to die in a few days, I want her at Wesley.

Remember almost a year ago I wrote and said I doubted Mom would see 89? Well, what do you know, tomorrow she'll be 89. She got through all that mess last winter and got on a really stable plateau for months. Now, however, for the past month, she's been losing ground. For the last week or so, we haven't been able to get much into her besides ice cream and juice. I made her a milkshake on Saturday, but she would only take tiny spoonfuls at a time. Oddly enough, yesterday when I was there, she was very much awake. It was mid-afternoon and I didn't try to feed her anything. It's hard to know what I'll find each time I go up there. Some days she's alert and others, I can barely get her to open one eye. If she was one of my Hospice patients, I'd say she's going to be checking out within a couple of weeks or less. But being Mom, I haven't totally ruled out the possibility that she'll bounce back to one degree or another for a bit longer. I'll keep you posted.

March 6, 2001

I called Dr. Tarkington this morning and told her what happened last night. She asked what I wanted to do and I said I'd like to put her on Hospice. I doubt putting her in the hospital would help at this point. She agreed. She said she'd start the paperwork right away. Then I called a nurse friend and she said it would probably take till Thursday.

Susan, could you call Virginia and let her know what's up. I will decide today whether or not I'm coming out – I probably won't – and I'll let you know when I get home from Wesley tonight.

March 6, 2001

We called Virginia & Bill tonight to fill them in. We aren't coming out. Gary decided not to come either. I had suggested we try to change my ticket over for Eddie to use, but he said no. Mom slept and woke every half hour or so today. When she'd wake, she was real restless. Hard to know why. I talked to the Hospice aide who will probably be her aide when Hospice kicks in. I've known her from other Hospice cases we've been on together at Wesley. Technically, there's not a whole lot they can do for Mom. There are no pain control issues or anything, but the extra TLC will mean a lot. Mom's needs are so few these days – just keeping her comfortable, moving her regularly, keeping her clean. When Tammy or Dora are working, I'm completely confident. But when they're off, we have different aides in all the time. Unfortunately, some of the contracts see a bedridden patient who doesn't move or talk as one who is easy to ignore. Now we'll have a Hospice aide, the Hospice nurse and a volunteer if I want one.   Happy Birthday to Mom!

March 8, 2001

Predicting Mom's time frame is difficult. Monday I would have said she had a few days. Tonite I'd say a week or two. She virtually hasn't eaten anything for 4 or 5 days except little spoonfuls of ice cream or milkshake. Even then, she either wrestles back and forth trying to avoid me, or lets her mouth hang open so the food rolls back out. She was awake a good part of the afternoon today which surprised me. I don't know where she gets the energy to stay awake. Mom's got tenacity and a strong heart.

CHAPTER 14

The end of the story

April 27, 2001

I attempted to publish Mom's story back in 1997, but without success. Michelle suggested to me that perhaps the timing wasn't right. I didn't know how the story ended. So now I know the end of the story.

Monday, March 5: I went in to feed Mom her supper, although she had barely been eating in recent days. She was groggy and not able to stay awake for more than a few minutes at a time. I took her temp and it was 102. I told the nurse and she called the nurse manager from another floor. She came and said she'd notify the doctor and asked if I wanted Mom to go to the hospital. I said no; I was sure this was part of the dying process. When I got home, I e-mailed my sisters to let them know and to say we probably wouldn't be coming out that weekend as we had planned.

Tuesday, March 6: Mom's birthday. I guess she fooled me; made it to 89 after all. Today she had a low grade fever and was <u>very</u> restless whenever she was awake, thrashing from side to side in the bed. I talked to Dr. Tarkington today and asked for Hospice. She said she'd take care of it.

Wednesday, March 7: Baby Sera was born, Susan's 4th grandchild. Mom was awake a bit more today. Perhaps she's pulling out of this?? She had one very restless spell and when I reached over to try to calm her, she felt as cold as ice. Then after a couple of minutes, her temp came back up to normal. I tried to give her ice cream, but she swallowed very little. Donnya was taking care of her and was doing a double and so had her for days and evenings. I went home assured that Mom was in good hands.

Thursday, March 8: Mom was very awake most of the afternoon today. Susan had asked if I have a feel for how long she has. I wrote them an e-mail tonight saying it is so hard to tell. On Monday, I would have said maybe a few days, but today I'm thinking it might be a couple weeks. Mom has a strong heart. Who knows. I pressed the social worker to get Hospice in ASAP. She said all the paperwork was in place and she'd call tomorrow for a meeting next week. I told her I'd be in tomorrow a little after 10:00 a.m. and I could meet with them then. She kept insisting on next week because she probably couldn't arrange a meeting that quickly. I kept insisting that she could.

Friday, March 9: The social worker called me at work about 9:00 a.m. to say that Hospice wanted to meet with me this morning. (I resisted the urge to say 'I told you so.') I arrived at Wesley about 10:30, greeted a few people and went down to put my coat in Mom's room. I was startled to find she had turned that corner into a vigil state, unresponsive, and I knew we were looking at a day, maybe two. I found out later from Dora that this change occurred sometime between 7:00 a.m. and 10:00 a.m. because she wasn't unresponsive when Dora left. Mom was lying on her back, breathing through her mouth, her eyes closed. She was working to breath. Her limbs were somewhat flexible, which is something Dora and Tammy and I had noticed occurred from time to time in recent weeks. Typically she was fairly rigid and contracted.

We went through all the paperwork for Hospice and the nurse manager said she would be sure that if there were any "regular" aides working the weekend, they would be assigned to Mom so we wouldn't have any contracts these last couple days. The only response Mom made was when anyone tried to clean her mouth. Clearly it was very painful for her. The Hospice nurse said they would order morphine for her to help the breathing and ease the mouth pain. Early afternoon, someone came over from Dr. Tarkington's office and said she was sent to see how Mom was doing before they ordered the morphine. She stood and looked at Mom for some time and finally said she had never seen her like this before. Well, guess what? Mom had never been actively dying before! She left with Ella (day nurse) and I assumed they'd get the medication. By the time the shift changed at 3:00, no medication had been brought. After 4:00, I asked Debbie (evening nurse) and she said she had no order for it, but she'd call the pharmacy to see if it hadn't been sent yet. They, in turn, said it hadn't been ordered. So she called the doctor's office, which was closed, and got the doctor on call. He said since he wasn't Mom's doctor, he didn't want to interfere and so wouldn't write an order. We went to a nurse manager next and she finally called Dr. Tarkington at home. She said she thought the nurse had sent in the order, but she wanted to talk to me before she'd call it in. She asked me how Mom was doing and was she in any pain. I said yes, she had mouth pain and labored breathing and finally she agreed to write an order, but not for morphine, for something else. (I was beginning to get the impression that this doctor's office had never dealt with Hospice before. This wasn't going as smoothly as most cases I've seen). Finally, about 8:00 p.m. they came in with some type of suppository medication.

At 4:00, Fr. Kennedy from Blessed Sacrament came to anoint her.

I got ready to leave around 8:30 and Dora said maybe I shouldn't go. What if she dies? I said I was pretty sure she wasn't going to die that night. Her skin color was still good, no mottling, she was still warm to the touch and there was no change in her breathing.

Saturday, March 10: 3:00 a.m. – got a call from Vicky (night nurse) saying Mom's breathing had changed and her eyes looked different. I got dressed and Gary & I went up to see what was happening. When we arrived, her breathing looked and sounded the same to me, but her eyes were open and glassy. I figured out later that the Hospice aide who came in to spend the night with her, saw a change in breathing as the medication was wearing off. She was seeing the labored breathing that I had seen all day Friday. But we stayed and I visited with the aide and with Dora through the morning hours.

At 7:30 a.m. we left to go to Mass. Then, I went home and slept for about an hour and went back to Wesley about 10:30. Things were about the same.

I tried several times through the day to get Mom to close her eyes. I'd put my hand right up to her eyes and they would close, but then they would just open again. It looked so uncomfortable. Gary came up about 1:00 p.m. with cookies for the staff. They were thrilled, as usual. About 2:00 p.m. another Hospice aide came in and said she could stay till 3:30, so we decided to take a lunch break. Before I left, though, Greg came in to see Mom. I had told the girls to let him know Mom was dying. He was coming in to work the evening shift over at Wesley Manor and stopped to see us first. He was always so good to Mom when he cared for her and even after his assignment changed.

I got home to discover that David had cleaned the bathrooms and vacuumed. What a great help that was! I got some laundry done and headed back about 3:30. When I got back, Mom's coloring had changed. She was very pale. Tammy had left and Dora had come in. I thanked God that Mom had only Tammy and Dora care for her on her last two days; her most familiar caregivers. I spent the rest of the day watching Mom, visiting with people, playing cards, doing my taxes. And I also took some time to pack up Mom's things and give things away. Dora said I shouldn't do that, but I knew I wouldn't be able to do it later. I took the kite, the rainbow and the pinwheel down and gave them to the girls for someone else. A little while later they called me into the dining room and showed me that they had put up all those things for everyone to see and so that "Bea will always be with us." I gave the little Easter rabbit in the carrot to Donnya for her little girl; the butterflies and the cat clock to Tammy, the floor lamp and the bear on the stand to Dora, the rabbit to Carolyn and the statue of Mary to Sue Howard for the chapel. I gave Mom's baby to Marion Mariotti, another resident who always fussed over this baby (and got exceedingly upset if I didn't treat it right) so that she wouldn't have to 'worry' about it any more.

Dora brought me some supper around 6:00 p.m. Early in the evening, Mom's breathing changed. It wasn't so much that she was breathing but rather that her lungs were just working because her heart was still beating. About 7:00, I started to notice Mom's face and extremities were getting cold. I saw some mottling start on her hands, feet and knees. I went and told Dora and the nurse, Ruth, that it wouldn't be long. They came and took a look and Dora guessed she'd die within half an hour or so. Ruth said no, she'd make it through the night. I said a couple hours. They left. I sat and waited. I was sitting in the recliner and considering dozing off when I had a sense that it was time. It was 8:40 p.m. I went to the side of the bed and said, "You're leaving now aren't you?" She pressed her mouth closed. Then she opened it and breathed a few more times. I said, "It's okay; you can go if you want. Go on with Dad." She pressed her mouth shut again, opened it and breathed a few more times. I said, "Go now. We'll be all right." She pulled her mouth shut a third time, it fell open, she breathed once and was gone.

Dora was across the hall and I went and told her Mom was gone. She hurried into the room saying, "No, she's not." She put her hand on her chest and said, "I think I feel a heart beat." I said, "No you don't, Dora." And with that, I knew Dora was as much family to Mom as I was. We stood there for a moment looking at each other and looking at her. It didn't sink in. Dora went to get Ruth. When Ruth arrived, she checked for a pulse, for a heartbeat and found none so she went to call the nurse manager. Meanwhile, Dora prepared to wash her. She got some warm water and washcloths and towels and asked for one of her warm flannel nightgowns. I helped turn Mom as Dora changed and washed her and changed the bedding. By this time, Ruth had come back and Dora asked her for a brief. Ruth said she didn't need one and Dora said yes she did. Ruth said no she didn't and Dora said she was putting one on anyway. It just didn't seem right not to. I agreed. We got her situated, straightened her legs, put a clean sheet on her and put a rosary in her hands. It still didn't sink in.

Carolyn and Maggie came in and the four of us just stood around the bed and talked about Mom and how it had been these past ten years. We picked out a set of clothes for Mom to wear and I put them aside for the funeral director. After a while, the nurse came and got me to take a phone call. We had to call the U of R to have Mom transported there for a brain autopsy as part of a research project she was in. The doctor there had to get my verbal permission to do so. He asked several questions for the record:

"What time did she die?"

"8:45 p.m."

"Where did she die?"

"Wesley Gardens Nursing Home"

"What was the cause of death?"

"Alzheimer's"

"No, the actual cause of death. Cancer?"

"No."

"Heart disease?"

"No."

"Pneumonia?"

"No."

"Did she have flu – anything!?"

"No, just Alzheimer's."

"That's pretty rare."

"I know, but that's what it was."

Then I talked Dr. Tarkington. She offered her sympathy. She was very kind and thanked me for letting her be Mom's doctor. We waited forever for the funeral director to call, and when he finally did, we made arrangements to meet the next day at 11:00 a.m. I called Gary in the meantime and let him know I'd be home in an hour or so.

I went back to Mom's room to get my coat. There she lay, her mouth slightly open, and a film had formed over her left eye, like a sudden cataract. I don't know why. I left as if it were any other time, any other day. It still didn't sink in. Why didn't I take in the fact that I would never come back in here and see her again? The routine of coming and going from the nursing home hadn't been broken as yet.

When I got home, I called my sisters and told each one, in turn, that we were now orphans. One laughed, as I did; one said she had the same thought; one said nothing. Such an odd thought, to be an orphan in your 50's or 60's, but there you are. Gary had called our son and daughter, his brother and close friends. I went to bed, trying to catalogue in my mind all the things I would have to do tomorrow. I wanted to sleep as long as I could and go to a later Mass, but that was a useless thought.

Sunday, March 11: I was awake off and on through the night and up before Gary. We went to 7:30 a.m. Mass, went to see Fr. Trovato afterward (what a kind man), then on to Wesley to gather Mom's things. I had given away a lot and would leave her clothes to other residents. She had mostly adaptive clothing for the bedridden and so they were a welcome addition from the staffs' point of view. We had to pick up her chair, however, and some pictures and things for my sisters – things they had sent to Mom over the years. I said goodbye to Jane, Mom's roommate, and then Gary rushed me out so I barely had time to say goodbye to Tammy or anyone else.

Meeting with the undertaker was an expensive enterprise. One of the curious aspects of it was this business of requiring a vault for the casket; just another way for someone else to get in on the monetary windfall. But when I asked how much it was, I discovered there were several prices for vaults. Why, one might ask – and I did. Well, *this* is the cheapest one, and then you can go up to the next level. This one has a guarantee on the seal, but it's not very good. And THIS has a really excellent seal that's guaranteed for life! Gary's question was, whose life and who checks on it periodically. I can just imagine how outraged all those poor souls are who were just laid in a wooden box and planted. We got the cheapest one ($650). And after all was said and done, we eliminated embalming, hairdresser, cosmetologist (closed casket), got the cheapest casket and vault and it still cost $5,824. $1,045 of that was for "Arrangements," which does NOT include transfer of the body, preparation of the body, supervision at the funeral home or Church, use of the funeral home or the hearse. $1,045 to meet with the guy for an hour???

The rest of the day was spent on phone calls and finding and making up beds. My three sisters were coming and my niece, Jacqui, and my nephew, Tim. Michelle and Andrew were coming too, but they would stay with David.

Monday, March 12: I decided to go to work today since our first 'arrival' was 2:30 this afternoon. I went to Church as usual at 6:30 a.m. and then on to work. I told a couple people that Mom had died, and when they asked what I was doing at work, I said I felt like I had to do something 'normal' for a little while, because nothing had seemed so in days. When I told Lil, I tried to describe for her Mom's last couple days and how I watched her take her last breath and that's when I broke down for the first time. But then, I pushed the reality of it to the back of my mind. Too much to do first – time enough later.

After work, I went to the cemetery to get the gravesite. The girl I dealt with was very nice and very sympathetic. She asked me if I wanted a double or single grave and I said single. Then she showed me the price list and there were single graves for $475, $550 and $600. I asked why there should be a difference in price and she said the mid-price was for the "Garden Sections," and the upper price was for the "Holy Family Section" (with a statue in the middle). I observed that all the deceased were in the ground and in Rochester, right? She agreed. I said we would be happy with a $475 gravesite. She brought a layout of the section and asked if I had a preference as to her location, and I said, "Yes, I'd like it as close to New Mexico as possible." That kind of momentarily took her breath away, but then she laughed about it. Later, as we were finishing up the paperwork and all, she pointed out the gravesite on the map and assured me she did try to get her as close to New Mexico as she could. Afterward, I drove up to see the section Mom would be in and found there was a row of trees and hedges all along one side. They weren't dotted all around the section like the "Garden Sections," but hey, it looked okay to me. Then I noticed that the trees and hedges were along the side of the road facing the "Garden Sections." I'm guessing that's so the residents in the poorer sections can't look across and see the "Garden Sections."

I've discovered there's a great deal of humor in this business of funerals. Unfortunately, those who run the show are laughing all the way to the bank, as they say.

We picked up Jacqui that afternoon and got her settled in. Later, she and I went through reams of photos to find some possibilities to take to the funeral home. David came over after work and right after supper, Gary headed out to Buffalo to pick up Carole, Virginia and Tim. Later, after they arrived, David, Jacqui and Tim went to get Susan.

Tuesday, March 13: We took our time getting moving and in the afternoon, went to Don & Bob's. This is a requirement whenever my sisters are here – and yes, we know it's actually Don's Original, but it will always be Don & Bob's as far as we're concerned. Tim and Jacqui don't seem to get caught up in all the fuss over D&B's, but then they were raised in Arizona and Virginia; what do they know? I'm sure they wouldn't recognize the significance of Abbot's either – although we didn't go there this trip as it was pretty cold out the whole week.

We had calling hours from 4:00 to 7:00 p.m. and while we made a pretty good crowd by ourselves, lots of other people came by as well, including two former school mates of Carole's. That was a real treat for her. And too, my sisters got to see most of the Farnan cousins whom they hadn't seen in years. Too bad it takes a funeral to create a family reunion. Another fun aspect of the calling hours was that David's girlfriend, Kelly, was meeting his extended family for the first time. We're pretty sure he coached her ahead of time, "No matter what happens, just keep smiling. Don't say anything; don't answer any questions; and if they make any sudden moves, don't try to run." Well, Kelly held up pretty well considering all the teasing she got. We've actually scared off many a would-be suitor to our nieces and nephews. We figure, if they can put up with us as a group, they'll be all the stronger for it. Fr. Trovato showed up toward the end of the evening and led us in some prayers and after everyone else had left, Michelle & Andrew arrived. They had driven in from Detroit and came right to the funeral home.

We went from there to a restaurant for dinner and generally kept the waitress on her toes the entire time. It takes a strong waitress to put up with the likes of us, but she was more than up to the challenge. There were 11 of us, and at one point, when there was an unexpected lull in the conversations, Carole turned to Kelly at the opposite end of the table and said, "So! Kelly!"

Everyone looked her way. She took on this 'deer in the headlights' look. "What exactly are your intentions toward my nephew?" Michelle whispered across to Kelly, "Say you're going to Ireland with us. Aunt Carole's been to Ireland. She'll like that." So, Kelly, who never lost her smile, repeated that, and indeed, it did seem to sway the crowd in her favor. Happy to report, Kelly is still with David, lo these two months later. (*Undaunted by our grilling, she married David in June 2004*).

Wednesday, March 14: The funeral. We got ourselves together and got to the church about 15 minutes ahead. A good friend, Larry Feasel, was serving as Deacon at the Mass. David and three cousins were pall bearers. After they brought the casket into the back of the church, Father sprinkled the casket with holy water and said the blessing. The four of us looked at each other with the same instantaneous thought in our minds. Mom's casket was covered with fabric, and we KNEW she was, at that moment, horrified that he was getting water spots on it. Well, we'll just have to deal with that in the next life, I suppose. Then the four of us put the pall over the casket, trying to get it as straight and as neat as she would have insisted on.

I had selected the readings and hymns for the Mass and Fr. Trovato gave a really nice homily, especially considering he never knew Mom. (The two priests I had considered for her funeral, who knew her, had both died in the past year). He even mentioned the fact that when the Deacon read, "In My Father's house there are many mansions," we translated that to "many Manions" – an old family tradition. We were all doing pretty well, actually, up until the end of Mass when Larry gave a talk. It was wonderful, so touching, so to the point – about end of life issues, faith and Alzheimer's. When he said, "Now she knows who you are," we all pretty much lost it.

From there we were off to the cemetery and as we stood around the gravesite, freezing in the bitter cold, watching the casket rock in the wind, no one seemed to notice that we were in the "poor neighborhood." We didn't linger, needless to say, and then headed back to the house for food, which our loving, talented niece and nephew-in-law, Nora & Mike, prepared and served. Unfortunately, Virginia and Michelle & Andrew had to leave fairly early because Virginia had to catch a flight out of Buffalo. Michelle and

Andrew were going to Detroit anyway and took her on their way. Relatives and friends stayed until late afternoon and we had a great visit. As the evening wore on, the rest of us just sort of grazed on the leftovers and sat around doing nothing.

Thursday, March 15: Two more of our circle left. Carole, Susan, Jacqui and I went out to lunch and then we took Susan to the airport. After a lengthy goodbye, Carole, Jacqui and I went to see the colossal Wegman's store in Pittsford. I hadn't been in it before, and we were all pretty well blown away by its size and variety of products. Jacqui got some little cupcake frogs for the kids and Carole and I got some half-moon cookies. We also hit a little Celtic shop in the plaza and then took Jacqui to the airport. Meanwhile, Gary and Tim had gone skiing.

When Carole and I got home, Tim was there and we decided to pop out to Pittsford Wegman's again so Tim could be amazed by it. He was, and he splurged on some fancy chocolates, some of which he gave us. (YUM!!) Then we drove down to where Carole & Terry had lived before they moved to Arizona and also by the house we grew up in; a little trip down memory lane. Funny how houses look so much smaller than you remember them.

Gary was just arriving home when we got there and we turned around and went back out to have dinner over by David's. He & Kelly couldn't join us for dinner, but they met us afterward for dessert since we were pretty close to his apartment. In fact, while we were waiting for a table at the restaurant, we drove over so Carole and Tim could see his place.

Friday, March 16: I had do an Alzheimer's communication and spirituality training session for a class of Chaplains. I had quite forgotten to cancel, so I thought I'd go ahead and do it anyway, and it turned out to be a good opportunity to take Carole along so she could see what I do. She seemed to enjoy it and took information on the class back to Arizona with her. Afterwards, we stopped by Wesley because it was right nearby. All week long I kept having the thought that I'd have to get to the nursing home on Friday after everyone was gone. Then I'd instantly remember, no I don't

– that's why everyone's here. But the thought kept coming back over and over. So we went. I ran into several people I knew and they were so sweet and sympathetic. Carole got to meet some of the staff and residents and see where Mom had spent the last several years of her life. I thought it would be really difficult to go in Mom's room, especially since they told me on the way up that a new resident was in there, but oddly enough, it wasn't. I went in to see Jane; the roommate wasn't in there at the moment; and I was really okay with it. What really touched me, and Carole too, was when Jane sadly said, "I really miss your Mother." Jane and Mom never spoke – Mom wasn't able to speak – but Jane was comforted just to know she was over there and that I'd be coming in on a regular basis.

Later on Friday, Gary & I drove Carole and Tim to the Buffalo airport. They were the last to leave and now we had to get back to normal. But what was normal? Normal was going up to Wesley four or five times a week. As luck would have it, there was a lot going on over the next couple weeks and I more than filled in the time, but that didn't ward off the sense of having to go there. My next trip to Wesley was on Tuesday. I still had a Hospice patient there and, of course, I wanted to see the 'two Janes,' Mom's roommate and my other friend Jane whom I had gotten to know over the past ten years.

I had very mixed feelings about going to Wesley. Part of me just needs to be there and part of me doesn't want to go at all. When I arrive, as I walk across the parking lot, I feel like I don't belong there anymore. It was my home away from home for ten years, but now it's just the place I go as a visitor. When I get inside, I feel at home, but then, sometimes . . . One day I saw Mom's baby in a chair at the end of the hall near her room and it struck me right to the heart. I wished I hadn't seen it.

On Monday and Tuesday, March 25-26, I went to Toronto for an Alzheimer's conference. One of the speakers was a former caregiver who told her story about her Mom and it was my story and I wanted to run down to the stage and have a long, personal conversation with her.

CHAPTER 15

Afterward

March 22, 2001

Here it is a week after everyone has gone and now I'm beginning to feel the change. When Carole and I went to the nursing home last Friday, it was okay. When I went back on Tuesday, it was hard. I ran into friends and they were entirely too sympathetic – I was no longer able to imagine everything was the same. I want to go back and do it over – do it better; even the dying process. I want to take in more of the experience, absorb more of her. From the day I took her to the nursing home, I always knew she'd die. Probably in a couple years, maybe three. With each noticeable loss of ground, I'd think, "Yes, this is the beginning of the end." But it wasn't. And nearly ten years went by and I never thought she'd really die. Then she did – and the ten years were gone in the blink of an eye, in her last breath. We can't waste any time, even when we think we have a lot.

It's going to take some time to realize this. I get restless every afternoon around 4:00. I dream about Mom; sometimes alive, sometimes dead; and I wake up every hour or so. 'This too shall pass.' I'm not worried about how low or how high I feel sometimes. I know the routine. I've worked with families in bereavement up to a year after they lose someone and I've co-facilitated support groups for Hospice. I've seen the patterns of grief and have been able to assure them all along the way that it's normal. And now here I am seeing this whole experience from the inside. Kind of weird. When Dad died, it was very different. I had some moments of sadness, but nothing about my life and routine changed because he hadn't been around for years. It was lots easier to think, "Oh well, he's just out there in New Mexico someplace." Onward and upward!

I found an old insurance policy of Mom's and I was reading it over. If it's still good, it's for $1000. I have to send it in with Mom & Dad's death certificates. Anyway, she took it out in May of 1946 and the application form is attached to it. Among other things on the application was this, "How often and under what circumstances have you taken aircraft ascensions?" Mom answered, 'Never.' Then, "Do you intend to take ascensions in the future? Give particulars." Mom answered, 'No.' Do you suppose this will negate the policy cause she broke her word? Maybe I won't tell Aetna that she ever took aircraft ascensions. Or maybe I could just say that it was after she had Alzheimer's and she didn't know what she was doing. What do you think?

March 30, 2001

Turns out Mom's insurance policy is still valid in spite of her having taken aircraft ascensions. The very nice woman at Aetna said I merely have to send in copies of Mom & Dad's death certificates, which I have.

Oh! And guess what? I got Mom's death certificate and it turns out that someone couldn't get it to Dr. Tarkington to sign it so they had the doctor at Wesley fill it out and sign it. He put in it that he "attended the deceased from 6/21/91 to 3/12/01." Interesting since he's only been at Wesley for about four years and Mom died on 3/10. Then, for cause of death he put; "immediate cause – congestive heart failure, 1 day due to arteriosclerotic heart failure, 1 year, due to end stage Alzheimer's, 2 years." Well, I've been on the phone with Dr. T, the Health Dept. and Wesley's medical office. The Health Dept. (after a momentary pause at my asking if I could change a death certificate), said either doctor can submit a change request. Dr. T said to get hold of the Wesley doctor and find out why he put such a thing on the record since Mom didn't have heart disease.

Besides being obsessive-compulsive about correct details, the other reason I want this fixed is because research centers get a certain amount of government funding and that is based on statistics. If death certificates show that the majority of deaths are from, say, heart disease, the heart research folks get the bulk of the government dollars. We need to encourage people to have their physicians list Alzheimer's as primary cause of death, or at the very least, secondary cause. It can make a big difference in how dollars are allocated.

April 20, 2001

Nothing in life is simple, methinks.

On April 3, I got a letter from the Monroe County Department of Law. It started out, "Please accept our condolences on the death of your Mother. While it is not our intent to intrude upon your grief at this time...." And went on to say that basically they want everything Mom owned – perhaps down to the clothes she is wearing in the grave. And if I don't cooperate, they will take me to court. "It is necessary that our claim be paid or, in the alternative, that an estate proceeding be brought in Surrogate's Court so that we may affect the collection of our claim." Also, I need to petition the Surrogate's Court to qualify for Voluntary Administration (?). If I don't do that, they will petition the court to administer the estate and "We would prefer that you take this action." They wanted an accounting of everything she has and, by the way, we already know what she has, so don't try anything funny! Various points of this oh so warm and friendly letter were in bold print and at the bottom in bold and solid caps, they said I was to submit the information IN WRITING. And under NO circumstances was I to call them. The point of all this was that they've (Medicaid) been supporting her lo these past 7 years and they want whatever's left. Okay.

So I wrote back the next day and told them exactly what I've got here, the checking account, the burial account, and pre-paid burial account, the insurance policy which I was checking on to see if it's valid. I said I would get in touch with Surrogate Court since I am, after all, already POA and Representative Payee, and if they wanted me to have yet another title, well fine. I was very nice. However, I couldn't resist the urge to add a P.S. "By the way, you might want to soften the tone of your threatening letter ... or drop the condolences and 'not our intent to intrude on your grief' line. They're rather incongruous, don't you think?"

I called the court and a very nice woman sent me an application. A couple days later I get this 4-page form asking for all sorts of info about all of us. I had to send a $1 filing fee, the 4-page form, the original will, a certified copy of the death certificate, postage paid return envelopes for each of the four of us and a copy of the Dept. of Law letter. Okay fine, so I did all that.

A couple days later, I get 4 checks in the mail from Lincoln Financial Group, one made out to each of us for $250. Not sure what to do with those just yet.

Three days ago, I got a call from Surrogate Court saying there was a problem. I'm not the executor. I said I know that but the executor (Susan) and her back-up (Bill) live in Arizona and since the Social Services people get everything, what difference does it make? She said we have to do this right and she'd send me two forms for you guys to fill out to 'renounce' your duties. Okay fine!

Yesterday I got a notice in my PO box that I had to pick up mail that had postage due. Guess who? Surrogate's Court! They took the postage paid envelope made out to me and stuffed everything I had sent them in it along with these two forms. No – correction – not everything – they kept the will. Now here's the best part. The forms read, "The undersigned … hereby personally appears in the Surrogate's Court, Monroe County and renounces all right to voluntary administration of the goods of the decedent." Well, if you could do that, don't they think you could be the administrator?!?!?! They know full well you live in Arizona. It's all over the stupid paperwork I sent them – and which they sent back!

Okay, so I tried to call our lawyer to sort this out, and he can't be found; vacation, I'm guessing. Then I decide to absolutely throw caution to the wind and actually *call* the DEPARTMENT OF LAW! I did and got an answering machine which said (I swear I'm not making this up) "You have reached the office of Estate Collections. Patty McNamara will be out of the office until Monday, April 23. DO NOT LEAVE A MESSAGE AT THE TONE. NOTHING WILL BE DONE ABOUT YOUR CASE UNTIL AFTER SHE RETURNS."

Okay, fine!! I'm sorely tempted to take everything to this Patty McNamara's office and tell her, "Here, you get in touch with my sister and do this all long distance. Don't try to contact me any further. Don't call. Don't write. I'm out of the loop." But I won't; at least not yet.

April 24, 2001

I finally got hold of people today and here's the scoop. I'm sending you forms to fill out for "Renunciation of Voluntary Administration." Even though it says you have to personally appear, they really don't mean it. The woman I talked to said you should just fill these out, notarize and send them back to me. I asked why they wouldn't go back to the court and she said, "Because you have all the paperwork," which, of course, as we all know, they packed up and sent back to me. Anyway, don't worry about the Monroe County part or the file number part. Just renounce and get them back to me.

April 25, 2001

On April 16 (shows you how distinctive this day was that I can remember the date), I experienced the first day since Mom died that I felt good all day long. When I thought of her, it wasn't with pain; and when I didn't, I didn't have this vague sense of a cloud somewhere in my brain. A whole day! The plus was that this made me realize that feeling normal all the time will happen eventually. For now, I'm just hanging on for the roller coaster ride. Sometimes when something or someone reminds me of Mom, I get really sad and just want to check out; quit volunteering and everything else and go lay face down someplace for a month or so. Sometimes I get depressed for no obvious reason. Then, just as suddenly and sometimes unexpectedly, I feel fine. The lows are getting to be a little less low and a little less frequent, and short of quitting my job, I do kind of throw myself into them to a degree. From all I've learned over the years with Hospice, if you resist the 'waves' and deny the grief, sooner or later, it's going to hit you like a ton of bricks and you probably won't even know why.

It's interesting, Susan, you mention that you talk to Mom and take her with you, so to speak. Carole said something similar. In one e-mail, she said, "I've been talking to her for so long at night, that nothing really seems different." Aunt Nan said she talks to 'sister Bea' too.

April 30, 2001

I think I'm going to send these insurance checks on to you guys. They're only good for 120 days and heaven only knows how long Social Services and the Surrogate Court will keep things held up. The woman from Social Services did say they wouldn't claim them, but I'm still a bit skeptical. What I'm thinking is that we should cash them so as not to let them expire, but not spend them till I get something in writing that this is legit.

May 2, 2001

I went for a blood test today and as the clinician was preparing the paperwork, she happened to mention that an aunt and uncle were coming for dinner tonite; they come every Weds. night. She went on to say that since she and her sister lost their parents, this aunt and uncle have kind of tried to fill the gap. She said she loves them, but she still misses her parents a lot. She still has a tendency to want to talk to them and tell them things that are happening in her life. I asked how long ago they died and she said 1981 and 1987. I told her both my parents are dead, too, and that Mom died just a few weeks ago. She said wasn't it curious that she brought up the subject just now. We compared notes a bit and came away feeling a bit better for it. I was able to recommend a book to her that I've just read, "The Orphaned Adult," by Alexander Levy. Interestingly, one of the things he said in the book is that you'll become unexpectedly connected with other adults who are 'orphaned' once you've lost both your parents. It doesn't seem to happen when you've just lost one parent.

May 8, 2001

After that Friday when I got that voice mail from Social Services telling me not to leave a message at the sound of the beep, I bravely tried again on Monday. Much to my surprise, I actually talked to Patty

McNamara. She said she didn't know anything about the court forms and couldn't help me. All that was between me and the court and she wasn't going to "go over their heads." So I asked about the insurance checks. She said if they were paid to each of us, they couldn't be claimed by her office. Before all this, she acknowledged that she had no idea who I was or about Mom's case because she gets "hundreds" of claims in her office. So I finally asked if she had gotten my letter at all and she said she had no idea. I told her she wrote to me on 4/2 and I responded on 4/4. She said she must have received it then, and also must have responded to me and that her letter was "probably in typing." My guess is that "in typing" means lost.

When I called Surrogate's Court about Susan and Bill not coming to appear in court, the woman there said, "Does it really say that?" I said yes. She said, "Read it to me." I did. She said to wait till she got a copy to see for herself. She did, and was amazed. Then she said not to worry about it.

This eventually resolved itself and the courts, Social Services and the insurance companies finally all went away and left me in peace. Paperwork, phone calls, hours and days of chasing around and all anyone wanted was for me to send Social Services a check for all Mom's money – which I offered to do in the first place, and which took minutes to do in the end!

May 15, 2001

It happened just as I predicted. I had told several people that my all-time favorite singer, Perry Como, would die this year and probably in May. And sure enough, he died last Saturday, May 12. Saturday night, I was upstairs when Gary called up and said, "Turn on the news! Perry Como died today! Just like you said!" How did I know? Well, he and Mom were both born in 1912. They were both married in 1933. His daughter was born in 1947 as I was. They both had Alzheimer's. Mom died right near her birthday this year. It only made sense that he would die right near his birthday this year also. His birthday was May 18. How sad for his family and for those of us who have been such ardent fans for so many years – and those of us who know what his family had to bear. His theme song that Mom and I listened to years ago on so many Saturday nights goes through my head over and over … "You are never far away from me."

POSTSCRIPT

Back on a March day, two weeks after Mom died, I wrote, "I want to go back and do it over." Do I really? The bad as well as the good? In the early days, when she lived with me, I knew nothing. I made mistakes, lots of mistakes that I wish I could undo. Now I know so much more that I've learned partly from 'experts' in the field, but mostly from all the folks I know who have had Alzheimer's. They are the ones who have taught me the most about how to communicate and how to care. Yes, I wish I could go back and do it over – only this time with the knowledge I have now.

If you read my book, <u>Alzheimer's and the Workplace</u>, you'll see there all the things I've learned since Alzheimer's came into my life. The main reason I teach communication skills and wrote that first book, is so that others just starting out can use these techniques and avoid some of the pitfalls that this disease can throw into one's path.

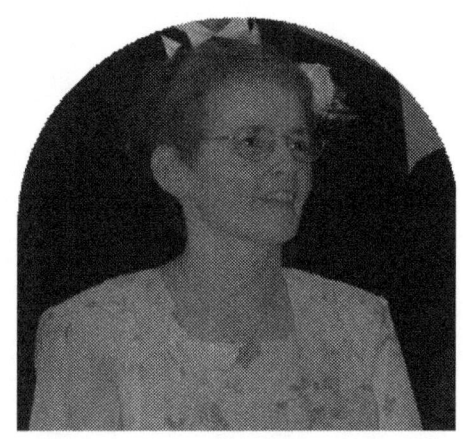

ABOUT THE AUTHOR

Born in 1947 in Rochester, NY, Patricia M. Thompson still resides there with her husband, Gary. They have four children: son, David and his wife Kelly, and daughter, Michelle, and her husband, Andrew. After raising her family, Patricia returned to college and obtained a bachelor's degree in Chemistry from SUNY Brockport. She worked in chemistry for several years, but over time, as three family members were diagnosed with Alzheimer's Disease, her interests turned in a different direction. Through various conferences, course work, and personal experience, she became proficient in the communication skills that are most effective in dealing with folks who have this disease. Besides caring for her own family members, she has been a volunteer with Hospice since 1986 and spends the majority of her volunteer time in nursing homes, frequently with Alzheimer's patients and their families. In 2000, she formed St. Colman Consulting, through which she offers presentations to police, clergy, nursing home staff, hospice personnel, as well as family groups and others.

Her previously published book is <u>Alzheimer's and the Workplace</u>. Copies of both works may be purchased from www.lulu.com/StColmanPress or from any of the online distributors such as Amazon, as well as from the author herself.

The author may be reached at pmtscp@rochester.rr.com